REFLEXOLOGY

NATHAN B. STRAUSS

Each part of our body is represented on the soles of our feet: Pressure on a particular point on the foot (a reflex point) affects its corresponding body part. The origins of reflexology date back over 5,000 years to China. Reflexology balances the energies in the human body by means of a gentle massage of the soles of the feet. Anyone who learns the principles of reflexology can use the technique of micro-massage to identify and treat malfunctions and energy imbalances in the body. While reflexology is practiced most successfully on the feet, it can also be applied to the hands. In this book, we present a simple method for utilizing reflexology (feet and hands). You can improve your quality of life, cure disease and alleviate pain and mental suffering in a simple and effective way. The book is richly illustrated.

Nathan B. Strauss lives in New York and is a physiotherapist by profession, specializing in alternative methods originating in the Far East. Strauss was involved in a traffic accident in 1987. In spite of extensive treatment, he did not fully recover. As a last resort, he began to undergo alternative medicine treatments which resulted in his complete recovery soon afterward. His personal experience and his professional knowledge motivated him to study and specialize in reflexology, Shiatsu and other similar methods.

REFLEXOLOGY

A Practical Guide

Nathan B. Strauss

Astrolog Publishing House

Astrolog Publishing House
P. O. Box 1123, Hod Hasharon 45111, Israel
Tel: 972-9-7412044
Fax: 972-9-7442714
E-Mail: info@astrolog.co.il
Astrolog Web Site: www.astrolog.co.il

ISBN 965-494-054-X

Published by Astrolog Publishing House 1999

Printed in Israel
10 9 8 7 6 5 4 3 2 1

CONTENTS

What is reflexology?

Reflexology, like other branches of alternative or complementary medicine, addresses the whole person rather than just a particular symptom or ailment. Whole or holistic treatment involves finding the root of the problem and correcting it, in this way alleviating or removing the symptoms. Practitioners of alternative medicine know that every part of the body – physical, mental and spiritual – is dependent on the other parts and interacts with all of them. In contrast to a consultation with a conventional physician, which is usually brief and centers around the specific complaint described by the patient, a consultation with a practitioner of alternative medicine takes about an hour, leading to a more profound understanding of the patient's problems.

There is an increasing awareness of the side-effects of drugs, some of which are not yet known; only time will tell if the drug is safe or not. Reflexology, which is a non-invasive, safe and risk-free therapy, does not rely on drugs for treating ailments: it employs touch in the form of simple pressure on the myriad reflex points on the feet or hands which represent every body part and organ. Thus, the whole body can be treated through pressure on these reflex points of the feet.

Reflexology can be defined as a stimulating mode of treatment, whereby a particular form of massage is applied to reflex points in the feet or hands in order to affect areas of the body which may be located quite far from the points themselves. While the hands can be used in reflexology, particularly for self-treatment and in cases where the feet cannot be used for some reason (such as infection or another physiological problem), the technique is more effective when applied to the feet, as the response to the pressure is greater.

Reflexology aims to rectify the elements which comprise the pathology of disease: congestion, inflammation and tension. In so doing, it brings all the body systems into balance and harmony. If there is an imbalance, it means that there is a malfunction due to congestion, poor blood circulation or tension. Reflexology breaks down tension, relieves stress, alleviates chronic or acute conditions, calms hyperactive areas down, and stimulates sluggish areas – such as the circulatory, digestive or nervous system – until the optimal balance between body systems is achieved.

Unfortunately, there are many factors that disturb the body's balance by blocking its energy flow: stress, worry, negativity, diet – and these present an obstacle to efficient body functioning. The resulting imbalance creates a build-up of toxins, preventing the free flow of energy without which the body will not experience harmony and well-being. By working on the reflex areas in the feet, imbalances can be identified and corrected, and an uninhibited flow of vitality can be released, restoring balance by triggering the body's inherent healing systems.

The history of reflexology

Reflexology is not a new method of treatment. It goes back thousands of years, to the ancient Egyptians and Chinese. In the Physician's Tomb at Saqqara in Egypt, dating from 2300 BC, there are murals depicting physicians performing foot and hand reflexology. The ancient Chinese used a combination of acupuncture and reflexology, a method developed by Dr. Wang-Wei in the fourth century BC. In 1582, two European physicians wrote about "zone therapy." However, the first real promotion of zone therapy can be attributed to the American physician and surgeon, Dr. William H. Fitzgerald, who began his research on the subject in 1913, following studies in London and a two-year tenure in a Vienna hospital, where he was introduced to the technique. Upon his return to the United States, he incorporated zone therapy into his practice – a bold move, considering the prejudices of the time! He discovered that applying certain pressures to the hands before or during surgery could lead to a decrease in pain. (This was significant at a time when anesthesia was in its infancy, and more people died from undergoing an anesthetic than from the surgery itself.)

Fitzgerald discovered that the body could be divided into ten equal longitudinal energy zones arranged symmetrically across the body, five on each side of a median line, and going through the body from front to back. Each zone related to one of the five digits on each side of the body – for example, zone 1 on the right side of the body begins in the big right toe, ascends to the brain, and descends via the arm to the right thumb – and so on, for both the right and left sides of the body. Each zone includes the body parts and organs that exist in it. Zone 1, for instance, includes the nose, mouth, throat, spinal column, and genitals, and is far and away the most sensitive of the zones. Fitzgerald claimed that by applying pressure to an area or areas in a particular zone, pain in other areas of the same zone could be diminished. To this end, he utilized clothespins, rubber bands, steel combs, ends of toothbrushes, etc., to apply constant pressure to the fingers and toes, and found that this pressure was responsible for alleviating pain in other areas of the corresponding zone. As the tips of the fingers and toes governed both the front and back of the body, they were considered the most effective places to exert pressure.

In addition, Fitzgerald determined that there were three transverse zones in the body, which were also reflected in the feet. Horizontal lines could be drawn (1) across the top of the shoulders (shoulder girdle) – which was represented in the foot by a line under the phalanges (toe bones), and governed the organs and body parts of the head and neck; (2) across the waist – which was represented in the foot by a line under the metatarsals, and governed the organs and body parts of the thorax and upper abdomen; (3) across the top of the pelvic floor – which was represented by a line across the tarsal bones including the talus (heelbone), and governed the organs and body parts of the abdomen and pelvis.

In summary, the foot is a reflection in miniature of the whole body, and the divisions are completely logical. If one examines the structure of the foot, it becomes clear that there is a system resembling a grid, and this helps determine the location of the reflex areas. As the foot contains 7,200 nerve endings that are linked to all body parts via the spine and the brain, it is an extremely sensitive area of the body. Each reflex area consists of numerous reflex points of minuscule size.

Fitzgerald found that if the foot itself suffered from some kind of condition, such as a corn, a callous or an infection, the pain increased rather than decreased as a result of the application of pressure. This continued until the condition cleared up. A further finding revealed that infections in one region of a zone not only affected the patient in that particular place, but led to pathological changes in some distant region in the same zone.

Fitzgerald's success rate was phenomenal for the time (sixty-five to seventy percent). He treated lumps in the breast, visual and respiratory problems, uterine fibroids, etc. His findings were published by Dr. Edwin F. Bowers, and while most of the conventional medical establishment scoffed at them, some practitioners were interested in the method, conducted research and made valuable contributions. One of them was Dr. Joe Riley, who introduced the "hooking" technique, whereby the practitioner's finger hooked a part of the patient's body and manipulated it. This technique could be applied to areas in the same zone as the area requiring treatment. Today, a milder form of "hook work" is used for massaging joint or limb areas in the same zones as the problem area; for example, massaging the lower arm in order to cure circulation problems in lower leg. It is also used on particular reflex points, such as the kidneys and the ileocecal valve. Riley had a chance conversation with physiotherapist Eunice D. Ingham at an orthopedic hospital in Florida, and as a result, she changed career direction and introduced reflexology as we know it today into her physiotherapy department. As a result of applying the method, her patients' pain decreased, their mobility increased, and their post-operative recovery rate accelerated. She established a private reflexology practice in the 1930s. One of her pupils was

Englishwoman Doreen E. Bayly, who built up a practice and established a training school for reflexology in Britain.

The possible mechanisms of reflexology

One of the reasons why reflexology is regarded with skepticism by some conventional medical practitioners is the fact that there is no scientific explanation for the effect that massaging a reflex point has on a particular body part or organ. Indeed, the mechanism is not fully understood, but it could be that the massage affects blood circulation and/or the nervous system. Healthy blood circulation means that nutrients and oxygen are carried to all parts of the body, and toxins and waste products are carried away from them, thus ensuring the optimal functioning of the body systems.

The reflexology massage may reduce pain because it releases endorphins (the body's natural painkillers) from the pituitary gland in the brain into the bloodstream. The energy that links the organs in the same zone has not been identified. When there is an energy imbalance in a particular body part, the aura or energy field around the corresponding reflex area in the foot will be weaker. (This has been proved by Kirlian photography.) Treatment with reflexology strengthens the aura, because of the improve- ment in the condition of the corresponding body part. Reflexology practitioners frequently encounter accumulations of crystal-like calcium granules in the reflex areas; these indicate an imbalance in the corresponding body part as a result of tension. As they are massaged away, the imbalance is corrected. However, there is not necessarily a crystal deposit for every imbalance.

The role of reflexology in stress management

The nervous system has a great influence on health; in fact, physicians claim that seventy percent of all disorders, such as hypertension, heart ailments and strokes, are attributable to nervous tension. The role of reflexology is to reduce stress and induce relaxation by stimulating the healing powers inherent in the body, leading to self-treatment and improved functioning of the body systems.

The negative symptoms of stress inhibit the flow of life energy through the body, thus depriving organs and body parts of vital life forces. The symptoms disrupt performance and diminish productivity, creating feelings of futility and frustration. They cause energy blockages for which there are no safety valves. As a result, negative feelings, fatigue, disease and tension build up. In addition, depression follows, undermining the immune system and causing illness and destructive feelings.

While stress is in fact a necessary, motivating force which per se is not harmful, it can be a very negative force if we are unable to cope with it. Most people need the shot of adrenaline that stress provides in order to do their best – in an exam, in a sports event, in a professional or cultural event, etc. However, when stress gets the better of us, our inability to manage it leads to the abuse of the body, and consequently to physical and mental disorders, such as disturbed sleep patterns, personality disorders and physical diseases.

Reflexology breaks the vicious circle of stress mismanagement by relaxing the whole body, jump-starting the body's wonderful natural healing processes, and treating the source of the disorder. It stimulates sluggish blood circulation, thereby facilitating the repair work performed by the body in regeneration of cells, and expediting the removal of harmful waste products that have a toxic effect on the body and cause disease. It restores the imbalance in the body's energy flows, and from there, harmony and equilibrium to body, mind and soul. As there cannot be true health without relaxation, this is the main therapeutic aim of reflexology. A reflexology massage can lead to the alpha state of relaxation – the suspension between sleep and wakefulness, in which the mind is emptied of all trivial preoccupations, and filled with serenity and tranquillity – the pre-requisite for effective healing. A state of well-being necessitates a healthy diet, relaxation, sleep and exercise. Moreover, it involves a whole new mindset regarding things that previously induced extreme anxiety and stress.

Stress need no longer be a threat. On the contrary: Once a person knows how to cope with it and manage it properly, he is confident and strong enough to meet life head-on, to maximize his achievements, and to increase his sense of well-being. He is in control of his own mind and his emotions, and this fact is fortifying and beneficial.

Administering a reflexology treatment

On the first visit, the practitioner takes a detailed medical history of the patient. This aids the process of treatment and also identifies any problems that could interfere with administering treatment – for example, corns or foot infections. (Certain conditions of the feet may actually reflect a disorder in one of the corresponding body parts in the same zone; for example, a bunion might be an indication of a neck ailment.) The patient should be ready to describe all previous medical disorders, diseases and procedures, as they have a direct bearing on the health of his whole being.

Some practitioners have the patient soak his feet in a warm footbath containing a drop of peppermint or lavender oil. This not only relaxes and cleanses the feet, but it cools them in summer and warms them in winter. The patient then is seated in a recliner chair, leaning back comfortably, barefoot, with his legs in a relaxed position, and his head high enough for the practitioner to be able to observe his face for changes in expression (a reaction to a particularly sensitive reflex area, for instance) or in complexion. The practitioner examines his feet, paying attention to texture of skin (an indicator of the body's general condition as well as of blood circulation), temperature (which is a good indicator of circulatory problems or glandular imbalance), and color (again, an indication of circulation). The practitioner takes note of any foot disorders, such as corns, tough skin (often a result of bad posture or ill-fitting shoes), blisters, fissures, verrucas, athlete's foot, swelling, scars, or varicose veins. An infection precludes the possibility of treatment, so as not to risk spreading the infection or infecting the practitioner. This is a case in which the hand can be treated instead. Varicose veins must never be worked on, as there is a danger of causing additional damage. Scar tissue can benefit from a gentle massage. Many specific foot problems can and should be treated by a chiropodist.

The general feel of the foot reveals a lot to the practitioner: a tense foot indicates a high degree of stress, while a limp foot can warn of poor overall muscle tone. Swollen ankles can be a sign of internal problems. Frequently, energy imbalances in body parts manifest themselves in changes in the structure of the foot.

Before the massage is performed, many practitioners sprinkle a bit of talcum powder on the foot. This absorbs perspiration, and also facilitates the progress from point to point. Oil must under no circumstances be used, as it makes the foot slippery, and the practitioner loses control of the tiny, highly specific movements that must be performed. The thumb is the main massage instrument, but often the fingers are involved, too. Usually, the right thumb performs the massage on the right foot, with the left hand supporting the foot – the top if the sole of the foot or any area "above the waistline" is being worked on, and the heel for "below the waistline"; and vice versa for the left foot. The thumb is bent, with the fleshy pad making contact with each reflex point, always moving forward. Short nails are a must. Not only does this position prevent nails from digging into the patient, but the thumb can move comfortably and smoothly from one tiny point to the next, always maintaining contact with the foot. The amount of pressure applied depends both on the patient's physical condition and on the stage in the course of sessions: At the beginning, the practitioner will tend to exert less pressure, in order to relax the patient, test his reactions, and become familiar with the story told by his feet. Usually the pressure ranges from 2-5 lbs.

The practitioner begins with the big toe of the right foot, working across the toes, down to the next transverse section (the metatarsals) and so on down to the heel. Then the sides and top of the foot will be treated. When this is completed, the practitioner may wrap the foot in a towel to prevent it from becoming cold. This procedure is repeated with the left foot. After the "detailed" treatment of all the reflex areas, each foot will undergo gentle rotation of ankles and toes, a "mashing" of the sole with the practitioner's fist, and a kind of "squeezing" of the sides of the foot, in opposite directions. The session ends with relaxing breathing exercises.

What is felt during a treatment

Some people think that reflexology will be unbearable because their feet are extremely ticklish. Usually, however, the practitioner's touch is firm enough for this not to be the case. If a ticklish sensation does occur, it may well indicate a disorder in the corresponding body area. There may be a "piercing" or "pricking" sensation (again, a sign of some disorder. The patient may be aware of crystal deposits being broken down. The more tension the patient experiences, the more sensitive areas he will have in his feet. The greater the sensitivity, the greater the imbalance.

Some sensations that may be experienced during a massage are: a slight ache in the locations where the energy blockages are being massaged; a "shooting" sensation as the blockages are released, followed by a spread of warmth; fluctuations in temperature, and jerky, twitching movements as a result of energy re-alignment; a desire to sleep; a euphoric state, and a feeling of floating as tension is released; a feeling of heaviness that comes with total relaxation.

Not everybody responds to the first treatment: Some

people are so out of touch with their feet, or there is such an extent of energy blockage, that there seems to be no sensitivity in them whatsoever. If the blockage is released, the situation usually improves and there can be a response to the treatment. If the lack of response results from paralysis or some other serious condition, continued treatments can improve the rate of response, demonstrating that some nerves are still sending messages to the brain unimpeded.

What is felt after a treatment

After a treatment, the patient is usually relaxed – often to the point of falling asleep! His feet will usually be warm. Some people are flushed and warm all over, while others may feel cold, because their blood flow has increased inward in order to heal organs situated deep in the body. A period of rest is recommended in order to enable the treatment to be as effective as possible in triggering the body's natural healing processes. While some people feel tired, others are energized, and full of a feeling of vitality and well-being as a result of fully-functioning blood circulation.

Reflexology has no unpleasant side-effects. At the beginning of the course of treatment, however, the stimulation of the body systems and the release of energy blockages may cause minor upheavals, which are basically manifestations of the body cleansing itself of toxins and accumulated waste products via the various excretory systems. As they are cleansing and purifying processes, they should be perceived as positive. In order to aid these processes, the patient should drink large amounts of purified water for 24 hours after the treatment. Typical occurrences following a massage are: frequent urination, with odor and color changes; increased bowel movements and flatulence; increased amounts of mucous and phlegm; increased perspiration, sometimes resulting in rashes; increased vaginal discharge, whose acidity may cause a mild irritation; changes in sleep patterns; recurrence of past medical conditions that were never completely eradicated.

Patients whose complaints have been evident for some time must not expect one treatment to miraculously cure everything. The treatment requires time, so several weekly sessions (usually six to eight) will be necessary in order for the body to balance up its systems and repair damage. The more serious the disorder, the longer it will take to treat. However, if a condition previously treated by reflexology massage should flare up, it usually takes a shorter time to treat than the initial treatment; if it is detected early on, it is very likely that the recurrence will be far less virulent. The length of sessions ranges from 45 to 60 minutes, depending on the sensitivity of the patient. The fewer the sensitive spots, the shorter the session.

The greater the person's faith in the healing powers of his own body, the greater the response to the reflexology massage. That is, the cure of disorders does not depend only on the number of massages administered or the seriousness of the conditions. It truly is a matter of mind/body/spirit interaction. The person has to believe that his health can improve, and that he is the one holding the key to this improvement. Moreover, with time, the person's awareness of his body processes will become honed, and he will have a greater ability to identify the cause of an imbalance.

Reflexology creates the correct environment in which self-healing can take place. One of the basic pre-requisites for successful reflexology therapy is the trust between the practitioner and the patient, and the discarding of all prior prejudices and fears concerning the treatment.

While reflexology is beneficial for correcting disorders, it is a wonderful way for a healthy person simply to enjoy a sense of well-being and total relaxation from the stresses of life. It is, in fact, a pity that most people seek medical help – either conventional or alternative – only when there is a malfunction in their bodies. It seems so logical that we should keep our bodies in optimal condition in order to prevent malfunctions and disorders from occurring, much in the same way as we take our cars in for periodic servicing, whether there is anything specifically wrong with them or not. Yet how many people maintain the balance in their bodies, or manage the stresses and tensions in their lives wisely, so that damage does not occur? Reflexology can help by building up the immune system and releasing blockages in the body systems, thus enabling the body to function at a high level of efficiency, so that health can be maintained. Reflexology can bolster the weaknesses in the immune system that cause allergies, recurring disorders, or viral attacks.

Reflexology treatments also constitute an early-warning system against incipient disorders by manifesting tenderness in the reflex area of a body part or system that is in danger of malfunctioning. Early treatment can prevent a serious imbalance or disorder.

In conjunction with a healthy lifestyle – both physical,

including exercise and diet, and mental, including relaxation techniques for stress management – regular treatments with reflexology constitute an excellent prophylaxis against disease, and maintain the overall health of the body. One hour of relaxation and massage of the reflex areas on the feet recharges the body's energy supply and ensures sufficient physical and emotional strength to cope with the ongoing demands of daily life. The sense of relaxation and well-being is definitely effective in preventing disorders.

How to make the most of this book

First of all, we will list and clarify the cases in which reflexological treatment (including self-treatment) must not be administered under any circumstances without the appropriate medical supervision. These include cases of cardiac disease, extremely high blood pressure, infectious skin diseases, blood clots (thromboses), extreme cases of kidney stones (or stones in the urinary tract), recent surgery (three weeks or less before the treatment), or pregnancy. In these cases, the patient **must** consult with a physician before commencing treatment – even self-treatment.

If during the treatment there is any occurrence of phenomena such as feeling bad, vertigo, fainting, pains, excessive perspiration, or a sharp rise (or drop) in blood pressure, the treatment must be halted immediately and a physician consulted.

When choosing between the reflexology of the hand and reflexology of the foot, it must be remembered that the treatment of the foot is easier and more effective, especially as all the points are bigger and more intensive than the points in the hand. Conversely, the position in a foot treatment, removing socks and shoes, and so on, can be problematic. The hand can be treated in almost any situation, but the points are smaller and it is sometimes difficult to locate them precisely.

While this book is meant for everyone, not everyone is a qualified reflexologist. Therefore you have to remember ten cardinal points:

1. There is no need to identify the exact location of the point that is supposed to help you. You can identify a broader area, in which the point is located, and even if you massage other points in the vicinity, no damage will be done – on the contrary.

2. Whole areas of the palm of the hand or the sole of the foot can be massaged, instead of massaging isolated points.

3. A general daily massage of the whole palm or sole of the foot is a prophylactic method against numerous ailments. This kind of massage is performed from the fingers or toes toward the root of the palm or the ankle.

4. The best massage is performed by using the pads of the thumbs. The fingers can also participate in the massage. When you want to press harder, clench your fingers into a fist together with your thumb (your thumb must be underneath your fingers), and use the outer flat surface to perform the massage.

5. The pressure of the massage must be felt, but it must not hurt. After a few treatments, you will learn the appropriate degree of pressure.

6. When you administer a general daily massage, you come across painful points on the palm of your hand or on

the sole of your foot. These points must be massaged gently for a few minutes, using the thumbs.

7. Do not perform a mixture of hand and foot massages. In each treatment, choose **one** of the methods and stick to it.

8. When you perform a self-massage in order to treat a problem, you should administer the treatment every two days. If the massage is general (prophylactic), it can be performed every day, but not less than twice a week. When you go to a reflexologist for a specific treatment, it is usually one weekly treatment (of about a half-hour). The longer you persevere with the treatment, the greater its effect.

9. In order to use this book correctly, read about all the reflexological points on the palms of the hands and the soles of the feet. Above each diagram, there is a description of the point and its location, as well as its use in treatment (professional or self-treatment). Below the diagram, there is a brief description of a case in which the particular point was treated. If you identify a disease or a problem which you want to treat, locate the point on the palm of your hand or the sole of your foot, and treat it. (Keep a detailed daily treatment record.) Bear in mind that the particular disease or condition can sometimes be treated via several points (on the hand or foot). Try all of them and, on the basis of your experience with the various points, choose the one which suits you the best.

10. The best reflexological method for improving the quality of life and for overcoming diseases and physical and mental problems is to start with a general prophylactic massage. During the course of this massage, you will discover painful points which will require an additional

individual massage; moreover, more points will be added according to the diseases from which you suffer (if any). After a time, you will have a "treatment template" which includes a general (preferably daily) massage, and treatment of individual points (preferably twice a week) which is tailored to your particular requirements.

This practical guide can teach you either to treat yourself with reflexological techniques, or to use them to treat other people.

REFLEXOLOGY OF THE HAND

The division of the hand presented in this book is into eight regions. Most of the points are situated on the palm. The other regions are the thumb (extremely important!), the fingers, the back of the hand, the root of the hand, the fingernails and the two "transition" areas. Altogether, there are 58 points. (Some of the points appear in a number of places, others contain sub-points.)

Fingernails

1

Point number 1 is situated on the nails of both hands.

If points number 1 are rubbed together, it helps combat dandruff, throbbing headaches and all hair problems. The most efficient method is to rub the fingernails of the left hand with the thumbnail of the right hand, and vice versa.

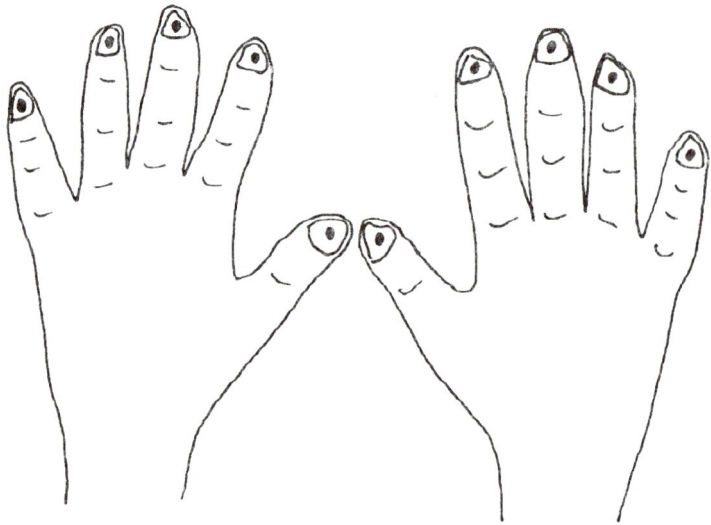

Tracy complained of headaches. We discovered the root of the problem completely by chance when she fidgeted with her braid and gasped with pain. Rubbing her fingernails decreased the pain, but we recommended that she change her hairstyle as well.

Thumb

2

Point number 2 is situated on the pads of the thumbs, in the shape of a hollow ring.

Pressure on the area of the pads helps increase concentration while studying, improve the memory, and relieve headaches.

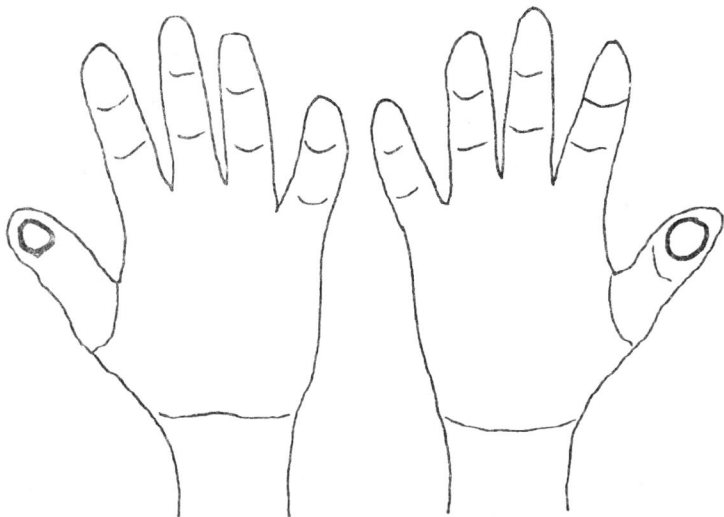

Martin, a student who worked and studied long hours every day, suffered from headaches and problems with his concentration. When he came to the clinic, he was on the verge of despair, as he was getting nowhere with his studies. After a few treatments consisting of light pressure on the thumb region for 10 minutes each time, he reported an improvement in his ability to study. He continued administering self-treatments twice or three times a day (and graduated successfully.

3

Point number 3 is situated at the base of the top joint of the thumb, under the pad, on the right side of the right thumb, and on the left side of the left thumb.

Pressure on point number 3 is effective for postural problems, high or low blood pressure, headaches and migraines.

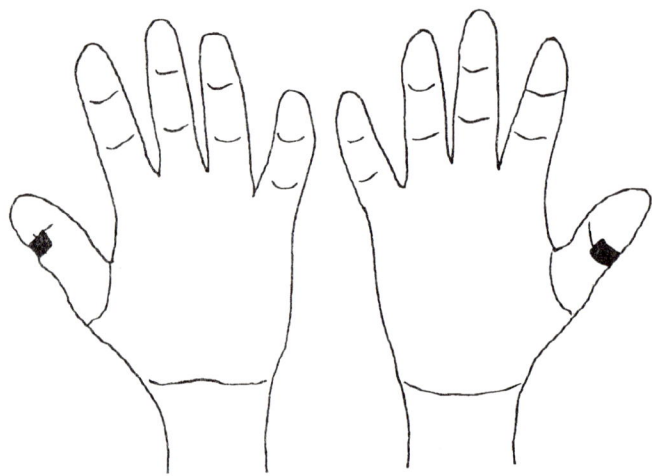

Sarah suffered from high blood pressure, which resulted in almost constant headaches. She learnt to administer self-treatment by exerting pressure on the appropriate points. (Because of the small area of the point, Sarah would use a pencil to exert pressure.) In the beginning, Sarah administered six daily 10-minute treatments. After the initial improvement, she decreased the number to four daily six-minute maintenance treatments.

After a series of treatments, Sarah reported that her headaches had disappeared totally, and that her blood pressure had decreased.

4

Point number 4 is situated in the center of the top joint of the inner side of the thumbs (surrounded by point number 2's "hollow ring.") Pressure on point number 4 helps in cases of depression, loss of appetite, schizophrenia, premature ejaculation, and hormonal problems.

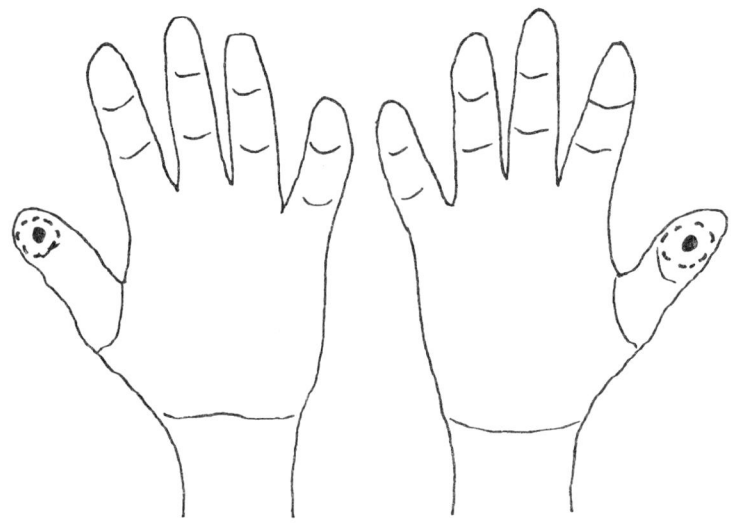

As a result of a tragedy in his family, Mike had sunk into depression, lost his appetite and become haunted by irrational and groundless fears. He arrived at the clinic in a state of restlessness and profound gloom. After lengthy treatment (due to the seriousness of his condition (there was a substantial improvement. He maintains the balance by administering two daily five-minute self-treatments.

5

Point number 5 is situated on the inner side of the center of the first thumb joint (opposite the forefinger), on both thumbs.

Pressure on point number 5 is effective in relieving pain in the temples, and for decreasing tension and agitation.

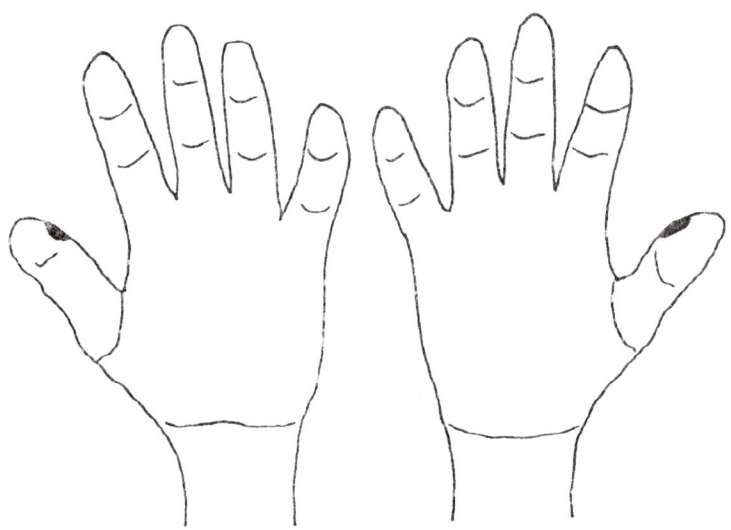

During the entire period of her divorce proceedings, Rachel suffered from pressure in the region of her temples as well as from extreme agitation. She learned to administer self-treatment about four times a day. After a week or so, she reported that she was back to her former self again.

6

Point number 6 is situated in the center of the thumbs along the inner side of the middle joint.

Pressure on point number 6 helps relieve headaches, vertigo, and impaired functioning of the senses (smell, taste, hearing and sight).

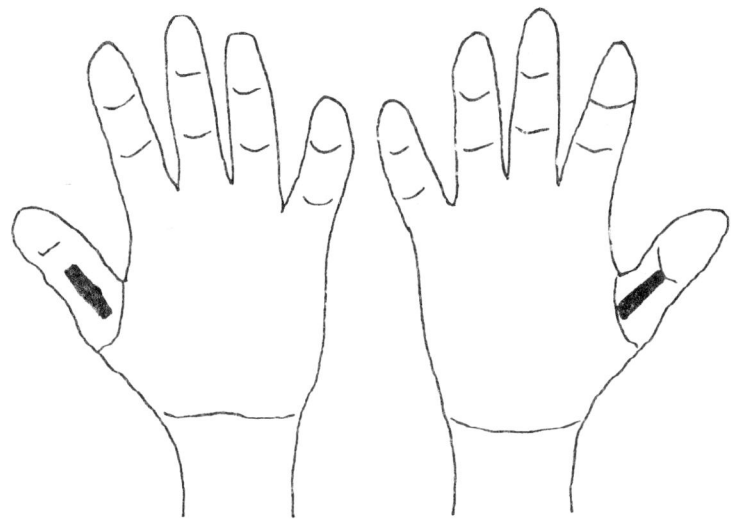

Daniel suffered from migraines, following which he would lose his senses of taste and smell. After he learned to massage the appropriate points, his migraine attacks decreased, and the loss of the senses of taste and smell disappeared completely.

7

Point number 7 is situated at the outer side of the top joint of the thumb.

Pressure on this point will solve nasal problems such as runny noses, nosebleeds, polyps, irritations and colds.

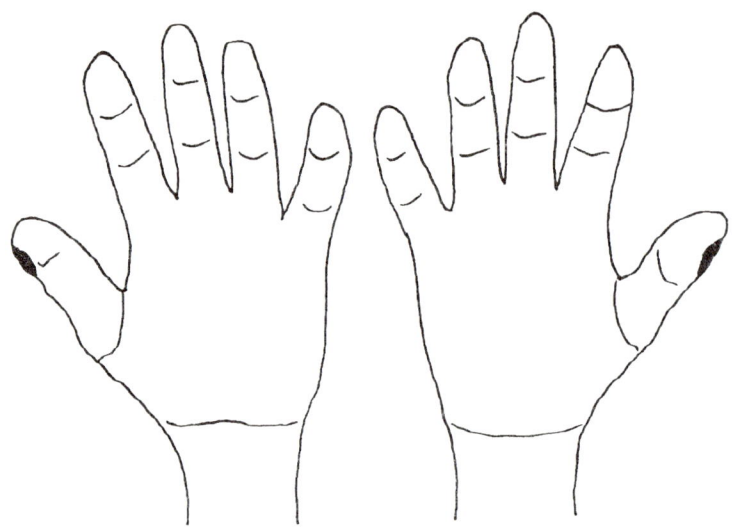

George suffered from nosebleeds and irritations of the nasal passages. The doctors recommended the surgical removal of his polyps, but George decided to try an alternative method first. After a massive course of treatment (four daily 10-minute treatments (the nosebleeds and irritations disappeared, as did the need for immediate surgery.

8

Point number 8 is a kind of strip which traverses the base of both thumbs (at the start of the bottom joint) on their outer side.

Pressure in this place is effective in cases of agitation, stiff neck and muscles, alopecia (hair loss), headaches, tinnitus (ringing ears), and mental stress.

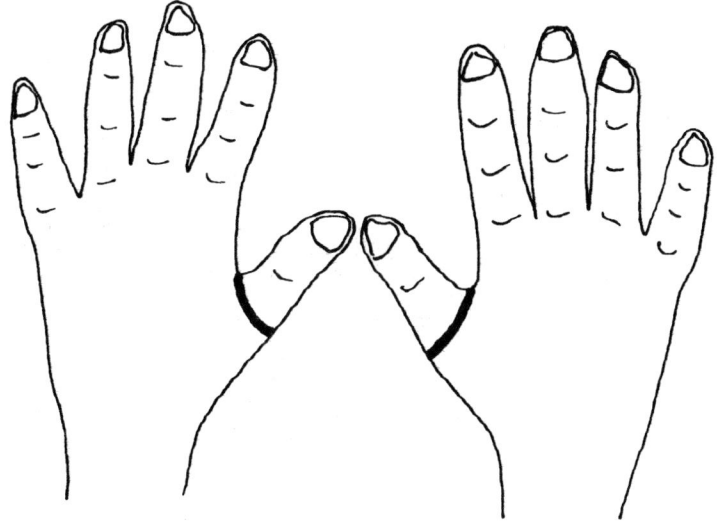

In Linda's job as a cashier in a large supermarket, she is forced to sit for hours on an uncomfortable seat with her body hunched forward in the direction of the cash register. She suffered from stiffness in the muscles at the back of her neck, as well as of the neck itself, and from headaches. Now she administers three to four daily four-minute self-treatments, and her suffering has decreased.

9

Point number 9 is situated in the center of the back of both thumbs, above point number 8.

Pressure on this point will alleviate toothache, receding gums, and pains in the jaws.

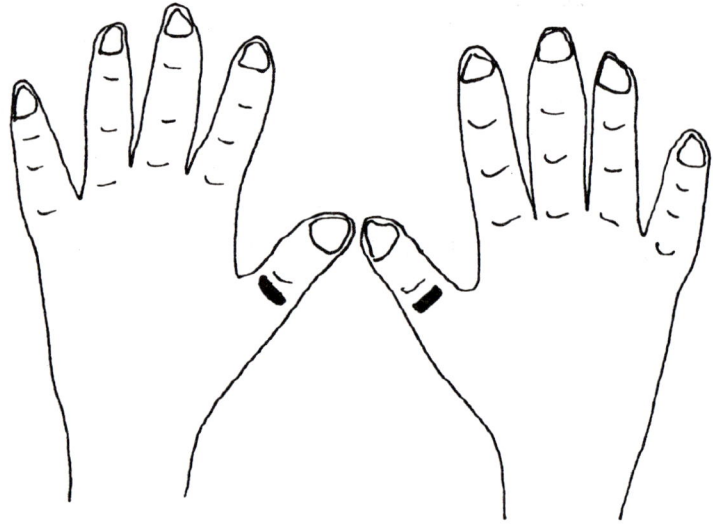

Carole was suffering from acute problems in the teeth and gums. Although she had undergone dental treatment, she experienced constant pains in her jaws. Ongoing treatments, three times a day for seven minutes each time, have enabled her to continue functioning normally, without undue suffering.

10

Point number 10 is situated on the back of the thumb, in both hands, under point number 9 (and 8).

Pressure on point 10 relieves sore throats and tonsillitis.

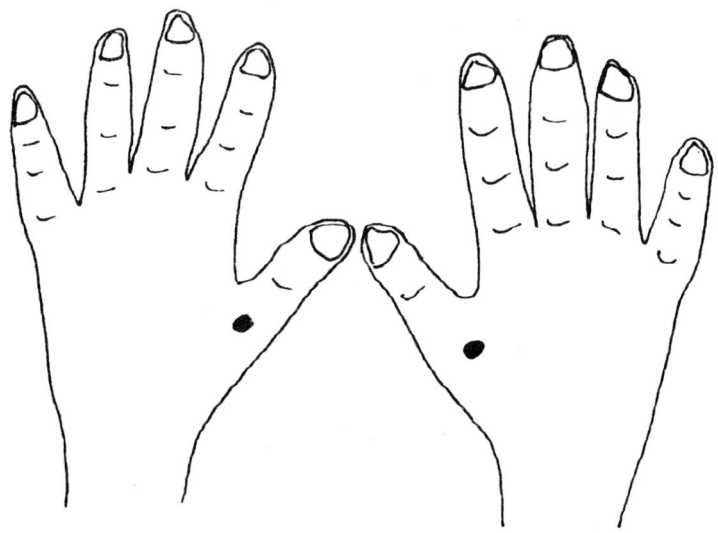

The members of the Ross family were very susceptible to throat infections, and often suffered from tonsillitis. After they learned to administer self-treatment by pressing on the appropriate point close to the base of the thumb, their problems ended. Each member of the family has his or her own daily regimen of treatment, ranging from three to five eight- to nine-minute treatments.

The Fingers
11

Point number 11 is situated on the strip under the index finger and the middle finger, and the space between them, on both surfaces of the hand.

Pressure on these points helps in cases of optical problems such as inflammations, near- or far-sightedness, night blindness or pain in the eyes.

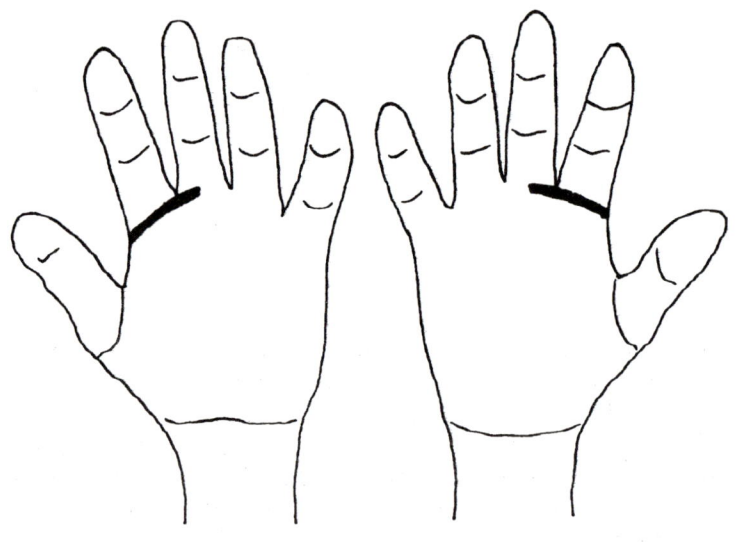

The first time Ruth arrived at the clinic one gloomy, rainy winter day, she was wearing darkly tinted sunglasses. She suffered from recurring eye infections, constantly watering eyes, and an extreme sensitivity to light. After an initial treatment and an explanation, she went home for the continuation of the treatment in soothing dim light. In order to facilitate the self-treatment, she pinched the area between the middle finger and the fourth finger eight times daily for five minutes, using a clothespin (switching hands each time). The infections and watering eyes gradually diminished, and Ruth administers a maintenance treatment to herself once a day for five minutes.

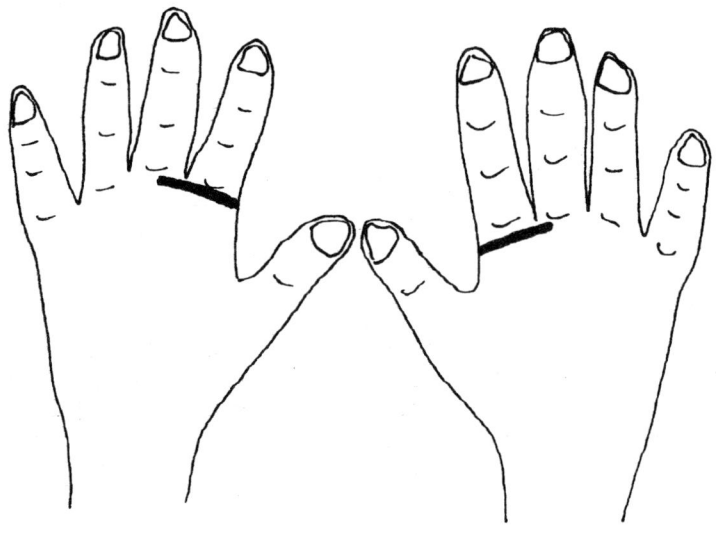

12

Point number 12 is situated at the tip of the top joint on the inner side of all the fingers and thumbs of both hands.

Pressure on this point helps treat runny noses, sinusitis, and headaches resulting from stuffy noses and sinuses.

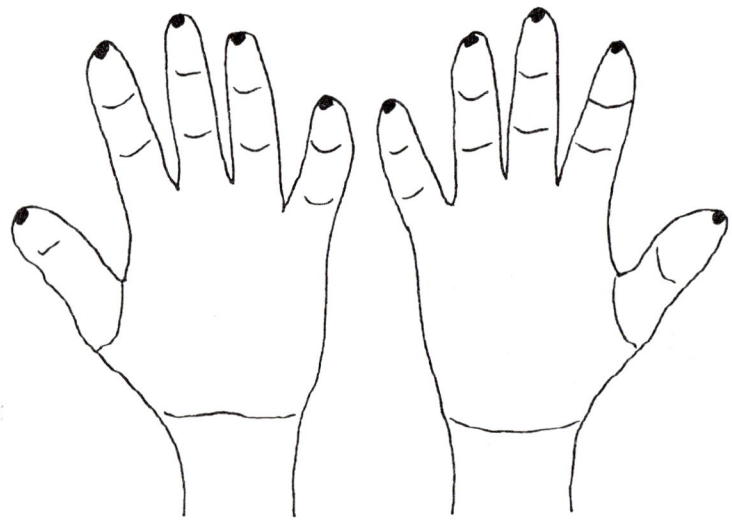

After years of suffering from a constantly running nose as well as from inflammations of the nasal passages, Simon came to the clinic totally skeptical about the likelihood of having his problem solved. The very next day (!), he reported that the stuffiness had greatly decreased. He does not go to sleep without pressing on all his fingertips, from the thumb toward the pinkie of the left hand, and then the same on the right hand. He hardly has to buy tissues anymore...

13

Point number 9 is situated on both palms, between the fourth finger and the pinkie, and under the pinkie.

Pressure on these points provides relief in cases of high fever, vomiting, toothache and auditory problems.

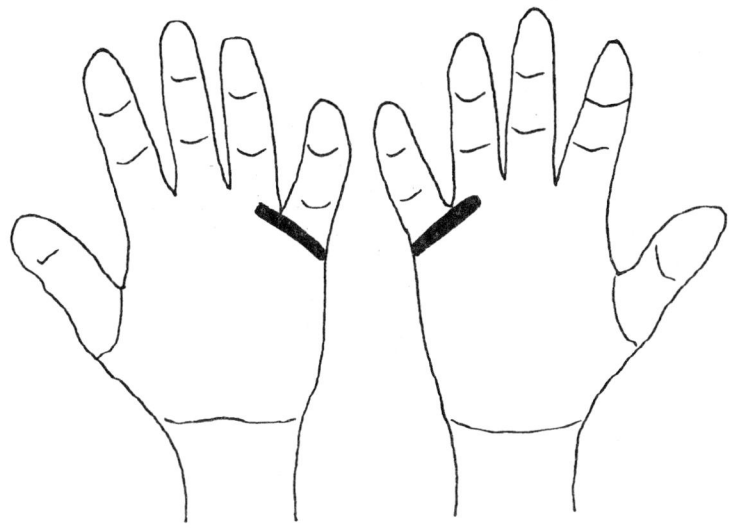

Barbara suffered for many months from an incessant ringing in her ears, sometimes accompanied by a sharp pain. After a course of four daily eight-minute treatments, her symptoms disappeared completely.

14

Point number 14 is situated at the sides of the upper joints of the index, middle and fourth fingers, as well as at the sides of the two upper joints of the pinkie on both hands. In the thumb, this point is situated in the lower half of the sides of the upper joint.

Pressure on this point alleviates any kind of pain, but especially toothache.

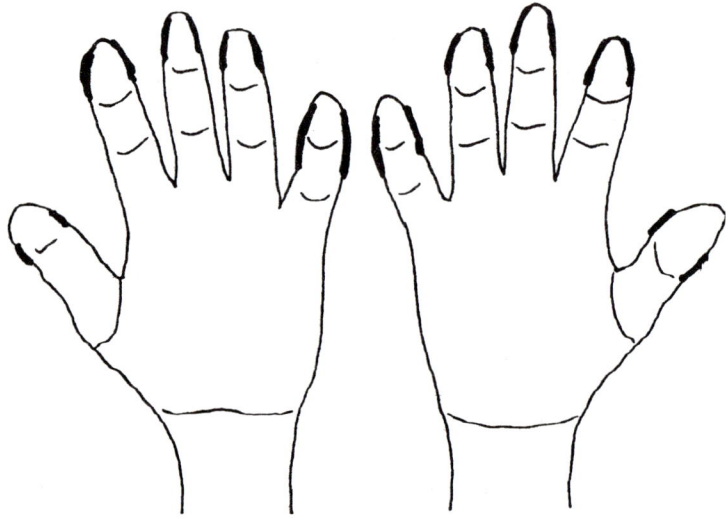

When you feel pain in your body, you should press on the sides of the fingers, starting from the thumb and going in the direction of the pinkie, first on the left hand and then the right. The treatment is particularly effective in cases of toothache, but is not a substitute for a visit to the doctor or dentist.

15

Point number 15 is situated in the place where the thumb and index finger are connected, around the base of the thumb on the inner part, as well as on the sides of the lower joint. The shape of the point resembles a crescent, and for this reason the point is called the "thumb crescent."

Pressure on these areas alleviates hoarseness, sneezing, anxiety and shortness of breath.

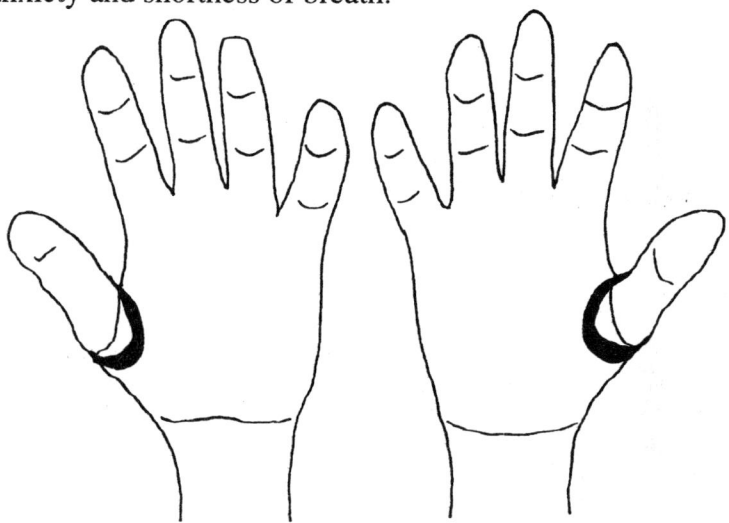

Abigail, a grade-school teacher, suffered from almost permanent hoarseness. In parallel, she was afflicted with sneezing fits caused by hay fever. After almost quitting teaching because of the worsening of these problems, a friend recommended that she come to the clinic. Now, after treatment, her symptoms have disappeared, but Abigail continues to massage the thumb region every few hours for five minutes each time to prevent a recurrence of the sneezing and hoarseness.

16

Point number 16 is situated on both sides of the second joint of pinkies on both hands.

Pressure on these areas helps relieve physical fatigue, lack of vitality, or problems of insomnia.

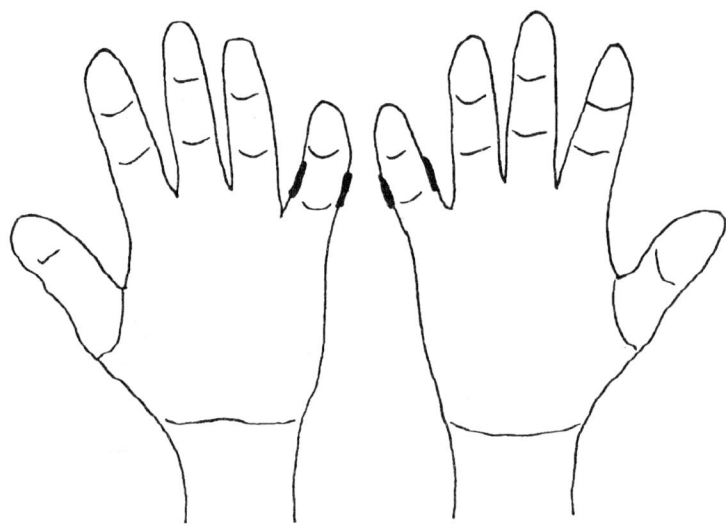

Jonathan, a 19-year-old soldier, suffered from fatigue all day long, and in spite of this, had great difficulty falling asleep at night. After he came to see me, at the recommendation of another practitioner, I taught him self-massage of point number 16 on his pinkies, three times a day for five minutes each. His problems disappeared completely.

The Palm

17

Point number 17 is a diagonal strip which starts from the tissue connecting the index finger and the thumb and continues in the direction of the base of the palm up to the middle of the "Mount of Venus" in both hands.

Pressure on this strip aids metabolism, and relieves skin and digestive problems.

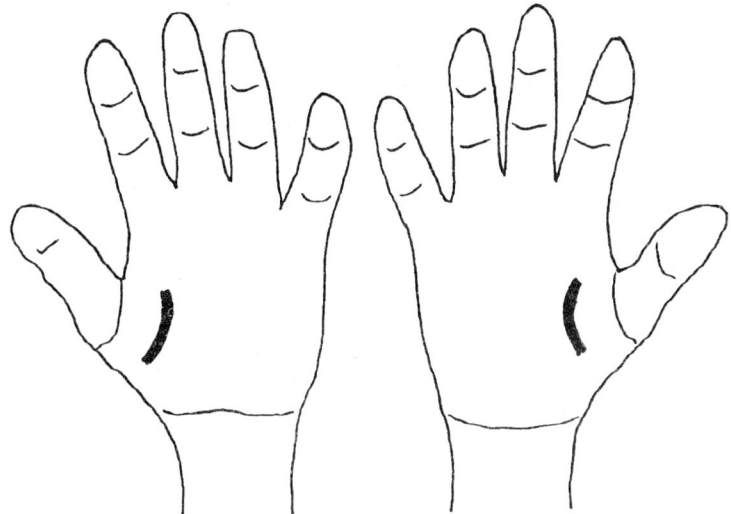

Roseanne suffered from an ulcer as well as from severe eczema on the soles of her feet. By administering three daily 10-minute treatments over a period of five weeks, these problems decreased significantly. Later, when it was discovered that she also suffered from osteoporosis (calcium loss), this treatment was effective in curbing it.

18

Point number 18 is situated next to point number 17 (in the direction of the center of the palm).

Pressure on this point is helpful in treating hypothyroidism and hyperthyroidism.

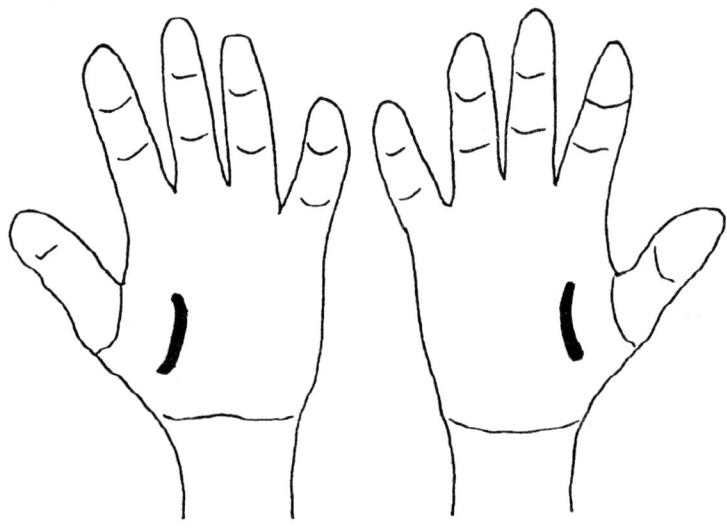

Alan arrived at the clinic with symptoms of a high pulse rate, insomnia and weight loss. After being diagnosed, he was administered four daily 10-minute treatments. About two months later, he stopped losing weight, and resumed a normal sleep pattern.

19

Point number 19 is situated below the tissue connecting the index finger and the middle finger at a distance of a finger-width on the palms of both hands.

Pressure on this point helps solve emotional problems, alleviates fatigue, and strengthens the immune system.

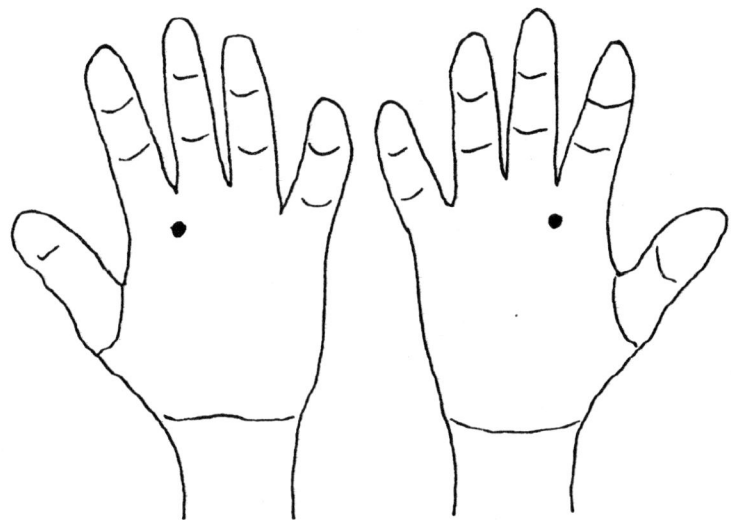

Following the death of her son, Martha stopped functioning. She no longer went to work, and often just lay in bed for days on end. After I had administered treatment to Martha during a few house-calls, her husband, Thomas, learned to massage her hands in the appropriate places until she revived and her vital energies were restored.

20

Point number 20 is situated below the **left** pinkie, approximately halfway down both surfaces of the hand.

Pressure on this point is effective in cases of cardiac irregularities, blood pressure and urinary tract problems, impotence, and prolapsed uterus.

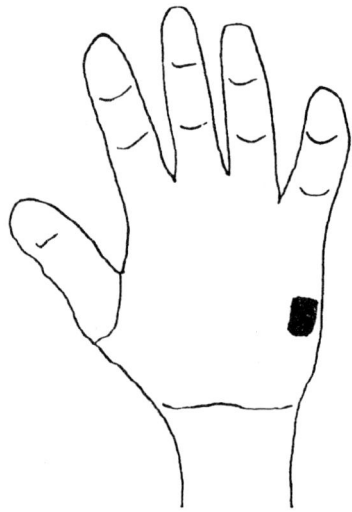

There is a history of cardiac problems in Celia's family. When Celia began to experience pains in the region of the heart, in addition to her already low blood pressure, she rushed to the clinic. Ten daily nine-minute treatments provided her with great relief. After some time, when she was receiving two daily one-minute treatments, she also reported that the bleeding she experienced between periods had ceased, as had an annoying cervical itch.

21

Point number 21 is situated on the palm in the region below the fourth finger on both hands.

Pressure on this region alleviates problems stemming from fatigue and tension, as well as balancing the nervous activity of internal organs.

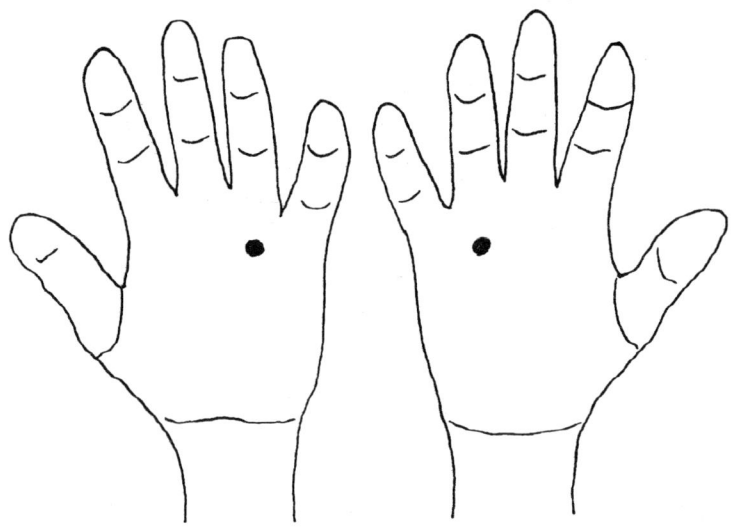

When Ray lost his job, he began to suffer from stomach cramps and partial paralysis in his face. He underwent four daily seven-minute treatments until his condition began to improve.

22

Point number 22 looks like a line below the middle and fourth fingers on the palms of both hands.

Pressure on point number 22 is effective in cases of breathing difficulties, flatulence, and pains in the region of the chest and diaphragm.

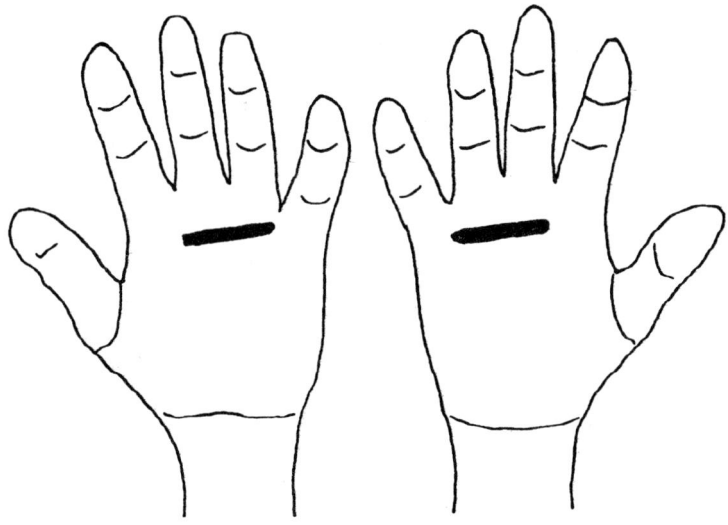

Gavin suffered from a nagging pain in the region of the diaphragm (not particularly severe, but constant. Medical tests did not reveal anything. A daily eight-minute massage of the appropriate point got rid of the pain.

23

Point number 23 is situated beneath the index finger in the region approximately in the middle of both palms.

Pressure on this point is effective for losing weight, treating problems of the digestive system, and alleviating nervous tension.

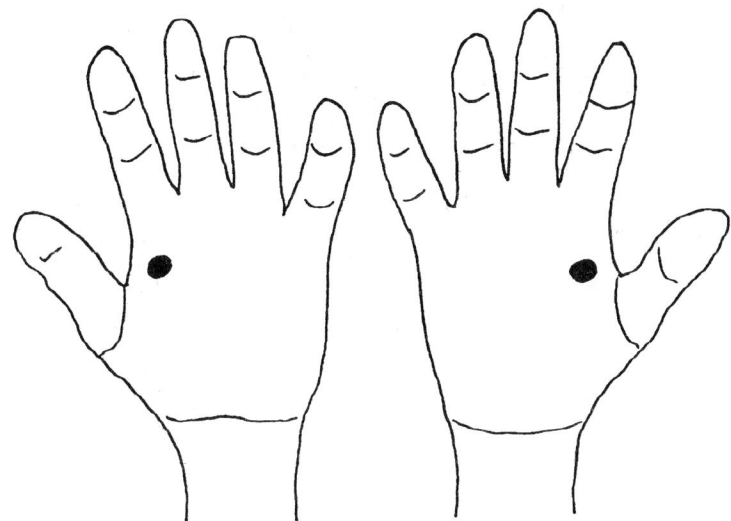

Susan was in the habit of calming her nerves by eating, and this was evident in her appearance. In parallel with an easy diet, she underwent a course of three daily five-minute treatments for several months. Now she is calm (and has a lovely figure.

24

Point number 24 is situated in the top part of the palm, at the edge of the region above point number 23, between the index finger and the thumb on both palms.

Pressure on this point is effective in treating diabetes, headaches, and malfunctions of the digestive system.

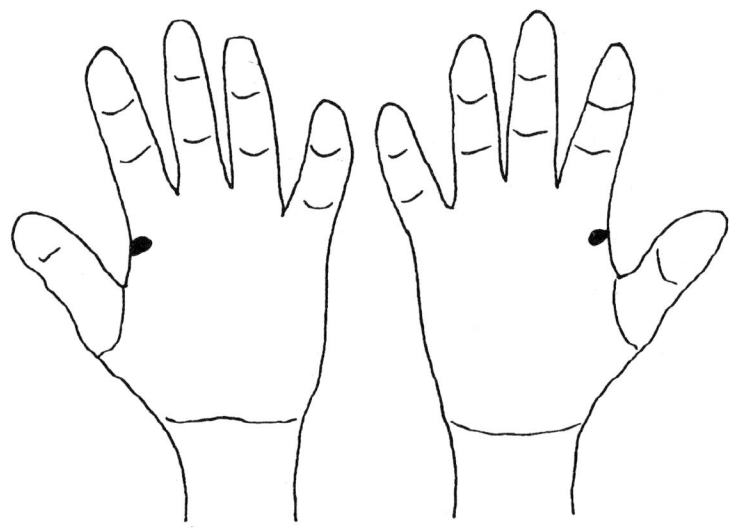

Jake suffered from constipation, resulting in headaches and stomach pains. When he got tired of taking various laxatives, he agreed to undergo three daily seven-minute treatments. Now he no longer suffers from constipation, and the other pains have also disappeared.

25

Point number 25 is situated beneath the fourth finger, approximately in the middle of the palms of both hands.

Pressure on this point is effective in treating diabetes, stomach pains, flatulence, allergies to food, and frequent colds.

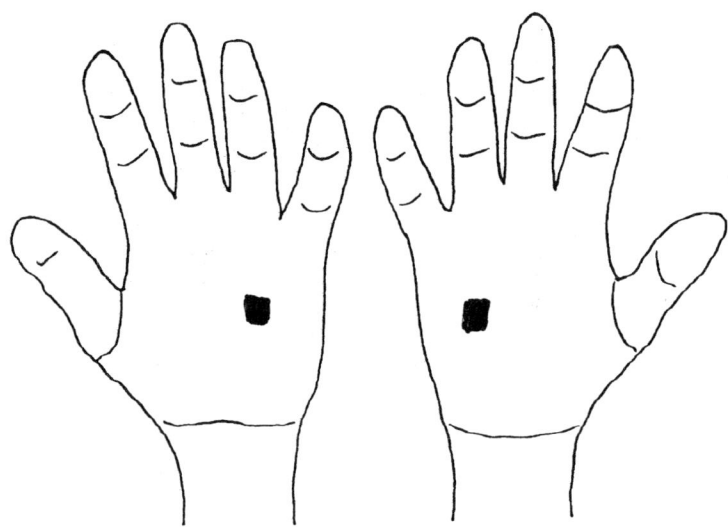

Sam was found to have diabetes. When he came to me, he reported a tendency toward frequent colds, excessive perspiration, and depression. We began with a massive course of 12 daily 10-minute treatments until there was an improvement in his condition.

26

Point number 26 is situated in the region below the middle finger in the lower half of the palms of both hands.

Pressure on this point is effective in treating ulcers, constipation, diarrhea and flatulence.

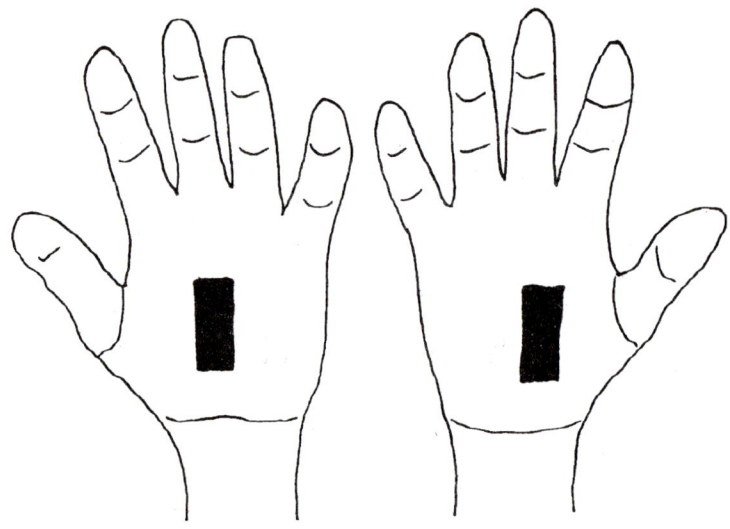

Jodie suffered from frequent attacks of diarrhea as well as from pains caused by an ulcer. The source of the problem was identified in the small intestine. A short course of two daily five-minute treatments solved the problem almost entirely.

27/28/29/30

Point number 27 is situated below the halfway line from the direction of the thumb slightly diagonally toward the center of the palm. On the right hand, the strip reaches the center of the palm (between the middle finger and the fourth finger), and on the left hand, it reaches the imaginary line that descends from between the index finger and the middle finger.

Point number 28 is situated on the right hand, from the center of the palm - continuing from point number 27 - to the imaginary line below the point where the fourth finger and the pinkie are connected.

Point number 29 is situated on the left palm - continuing from point number 27 - from the imaginary line that descends to the center from the point where the index finger and the middle finger are connected.

Point number 30 is situated on the left palm, from the center to the imaginary line below the point where the fourth finger and the pinkie are connected, beneath the halfway line.

Pressure on points number 27, 28, 29 and 30 helps solve problems in the digestive system.

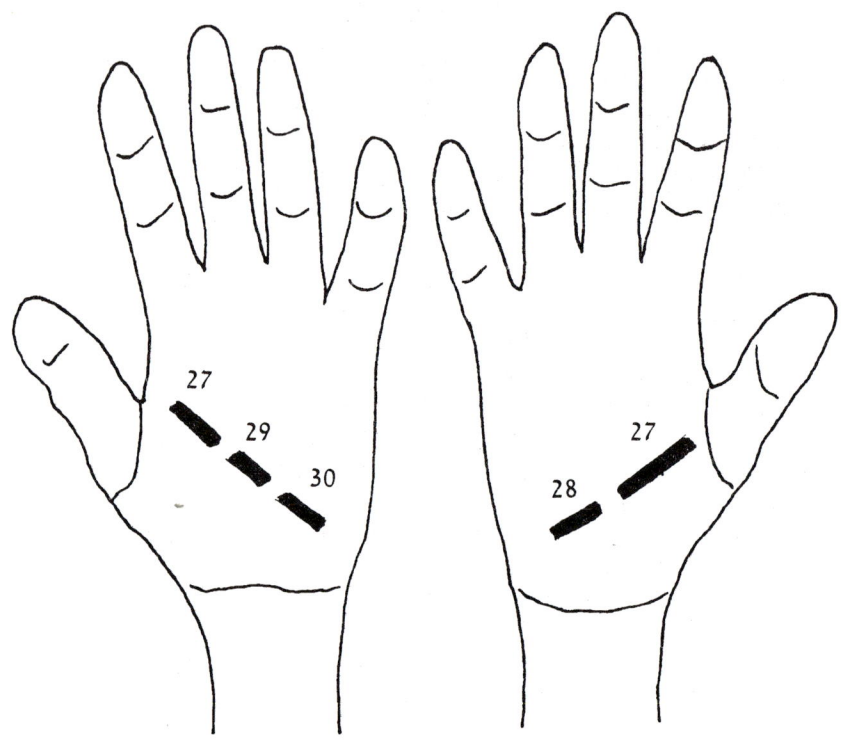

It is recommended that most people who come to the clinic with digestive problems stemming from the large intestine (mainly abdominal pains and constipation) undergo a course of two to four daily five to six-minute treatments on *each* of the four points. All the patients report varying degrees of improvement.

31

Point number 31 is situated on the imaginary vertical line that descends from the pinkie to the lower half of the **left** palm. In fact, point number 31 is situated at the end of point number 30.

Pressure on this point helps solve problems of anal control, inflammations and hemorrhoids.

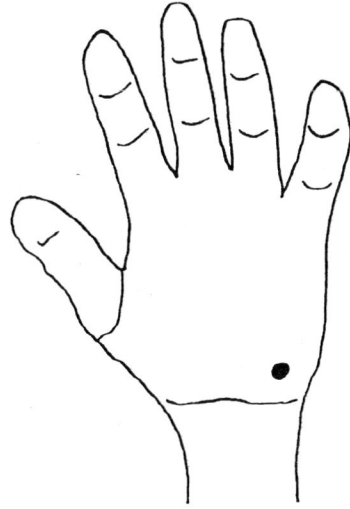

As a result of a boil in the anus, Chris was no longer able to control his rectal muscles, much to his own and other people's discomfort. The care-giver in the senior citizens' home where he lived knew how to press the appropriate point on his left palm three times a day, which eventually eliminated the need for extra diaper changes.

32

Point number 32 is situated above the root of the palm and the back of both hands, and it is a big, broad point.

Pressure on this point provides relief in cases of muscle spasms, varicose veins, ambulatory difficulties, and almost any problem in the lower part of the body.

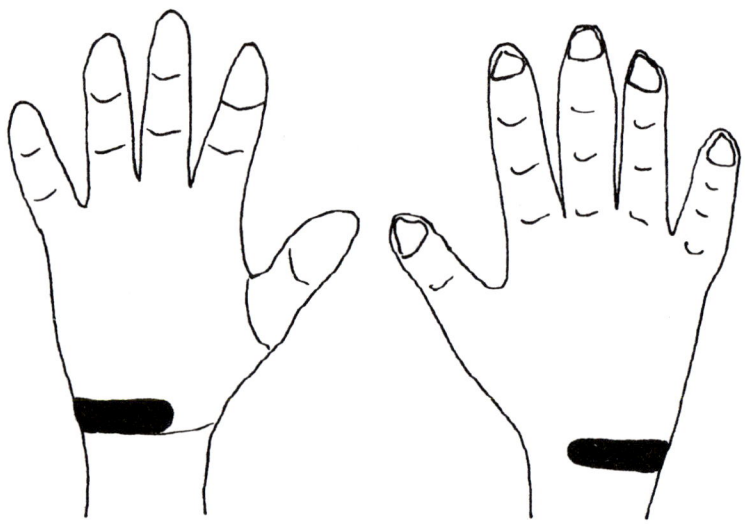

After completing his tour of duty in the military, Jason discovered that his legs weren't what they used to be. He had trouble walking long distances, developed ugly, painful veins, and suffered from frequent muscle spasms. In short, this was not how a young, newly discharged soldier should feel. His condition was gradually alleviated by means of six daily seven-minute treatments.

33

Point number 33 is situated on the palms in the region below the middle finger, in the upper part of the palm. Pressure on this point is effective in treating problems of the immune system, diabetes, weak nerves, and hormonal problems.

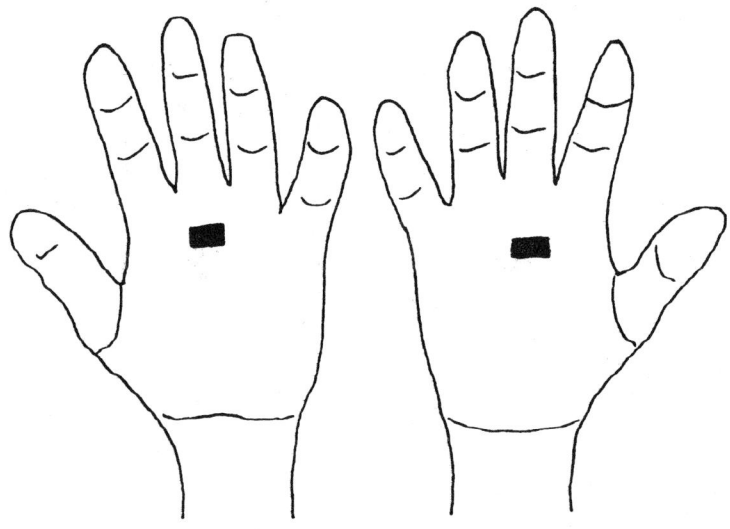

Twelve daily 10-minute treatments over the period of a year helped Betty return to normal after months of unexplained fainting spells, vomiting, irregular periods, and anger at the whole world.

34

Point number 34 is situated below point number 33 on the palms of both hands.

Pressure on this point is effective in all kidney problems, liver problems, red face and nose, lack of virility as a result of anxiety, bronchitis, asthma, and fainting spells.

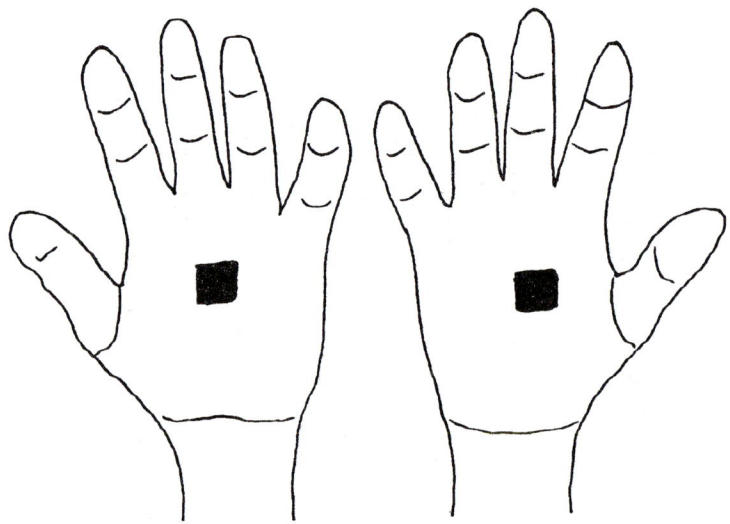

Tammy discovered that she was urinating frequently and heavily, and her feet tended to "fall asleep" often. Len came to the clinic because of his flushed face and prolonged erection. The symptoms of both patients indicated the need to treat the point that is connected to the kidney. The maximum course of 14 daily nine-minute treatments helped, and eventually each patient continued with the number of treatments appropriate to his or her condition.

35

Point number 35 is situated halfway down the palm and downward (in the direction of the root) along the imaginary line between the middle and fourth fingers.

Pressure on this point from top to bottom makes urination easier and is helpful in cases of urinary tract infections.

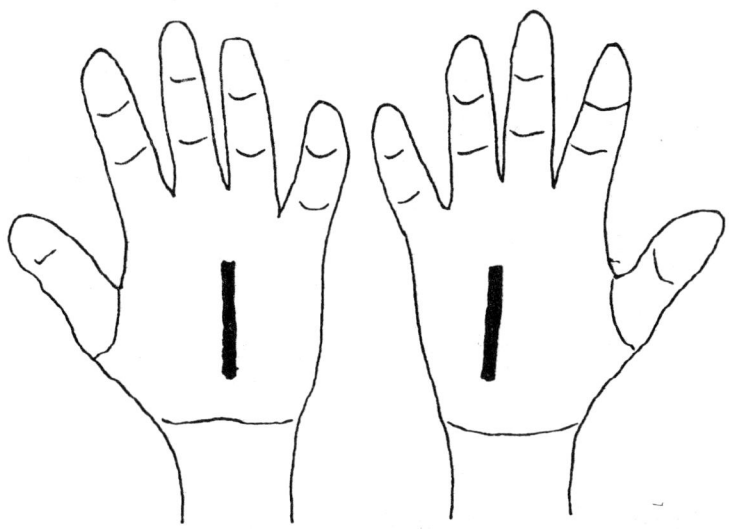

Renee suffered from recurring urinary tract infections. Three daily six-minute treatments sufficed to cause the pain and infection to disappear.

36

Point number 36 is situated between point number 35 and the root of the palm, and it is broader than point number 35.

Pressure on this point alleviates urinary tract infections, painful urination, and bed-wetting in children.

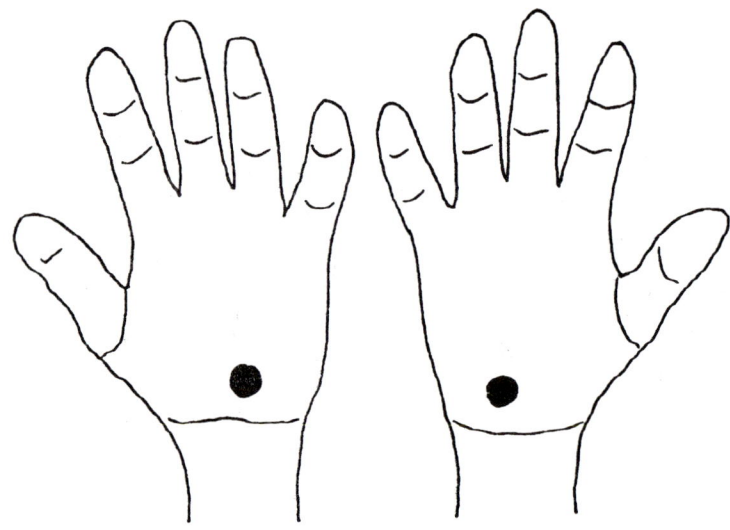

At the beginning of first grade, Peter, my neighbor's son, was still wetting his bed. After it had been determined that there were no psychological grounds for this, and when pre-bedtime urinating did not help, I recommended that the parents administer three daily six-minute massages to the appropriate point on the hand. Now Peter's sheets no longer flap in the breeze every day...

37

Point number 37 is situated below the index finger in the upper half of both palms.

Pressure on this point is effective in treating inflammations, swollen glands and lymphatic infections in the upper part of the body.

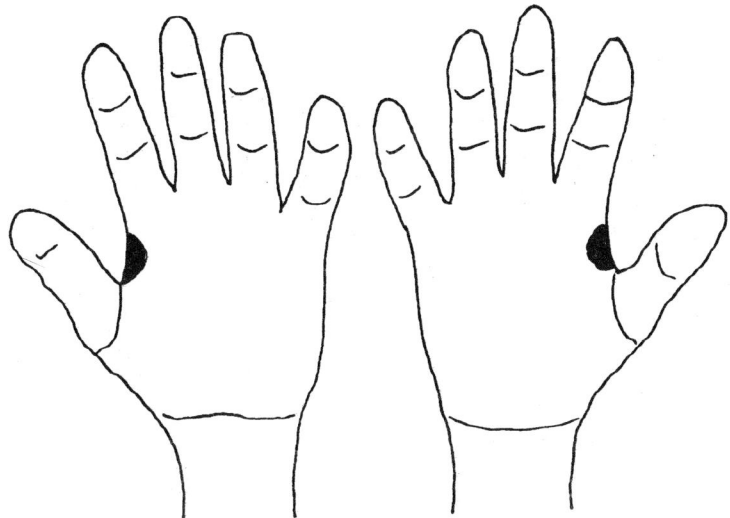

38

Point number 38 is situated below the pinkie, on the edge of both palms.

Pressure on this point is helpful in treating inflammations, swollen glands and lymphatic infections in the lower part of the body.

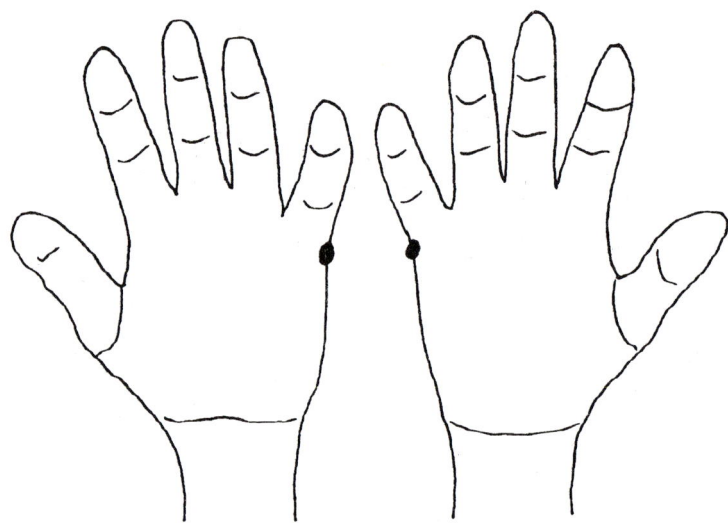

Lymphatic inflammations and glandular infections created painful sensitivity in various parts of Earl's body. A lengthy course of nine daily five-minute massages caused the swelling and pain to disappear.

39

Point number 39 is situated on the palm, on the line that descends from the space between the pinkie and the fourth finger, halfway to the root of the palm. The point is mainly felt in the right hand.

Pressure on this point helps to alleviate inflammations of the intestines (mainly "hidden" inflammations in the connecting passages between the small intestine and the large intestine).

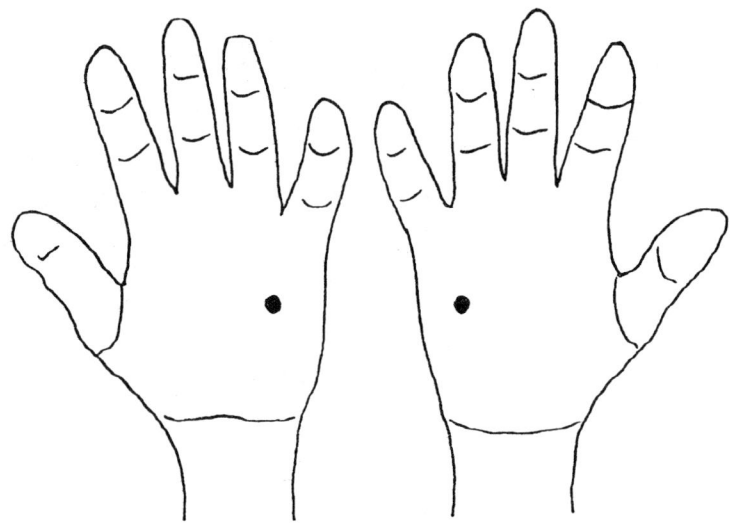

John suffered from intestinal cramps and painful stomach-aches, without any apparent medical reason. A course of five strong three-minute treatments on this point solved the problem.

40

Point number 40 is situated below point number 39. It is small, and is mainly felt in the right hand, and is usually treated together with point number 39.

Pressure on this point solves problems of gas in the digestive tract, appendicitis-like pains, and appendicitis.

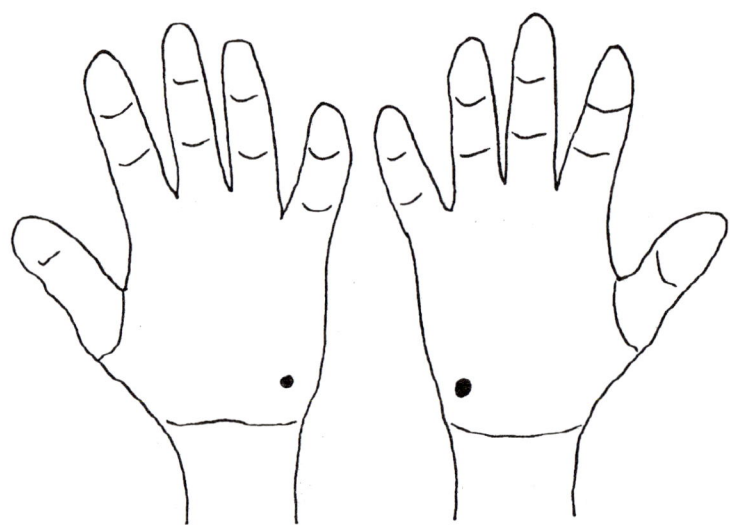

Shirley suffered from flatulence, she broke wind incessantly, although nothing in her diet could account for this. Ten to twelve daily three-minute treatments for three consecutive days solved her problem and made life for the people around her more pleasant.

41

Point number 41 (known as "the king's point," as it is "the solution to every problem") is situated on the edges of the lower joint of the thumb, which constitutes the major part of the "Mount of Venus" on the palm. (This point protrudes to such an extent that even on the back of the hand, in the corresponding place, it can be felt and treated.)

Pressure on this point is good for treating almost anything, and is used in many cases as a "rescue point," when the ailment of the patient cannot be identified. In any event, two daily five-minute treatments of this point improve the person's health.

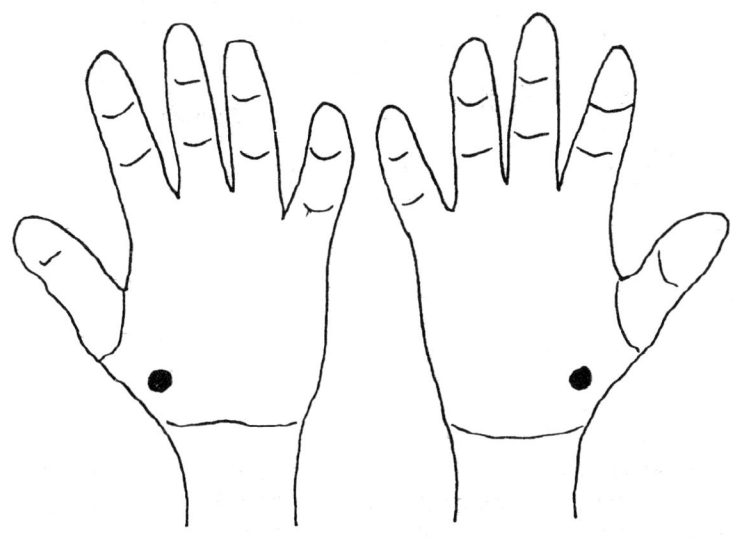

The Palm/The Back of the Hand
42

Point number 42 is situated on both surfaces of the hand in the region below the middle finger and the fourth finger, in the upper quarter of the hand.

Pressure on these points helps in treating asthma, pneumonia, anorexia, vertigo, and mastalgia (pains in the breasts).

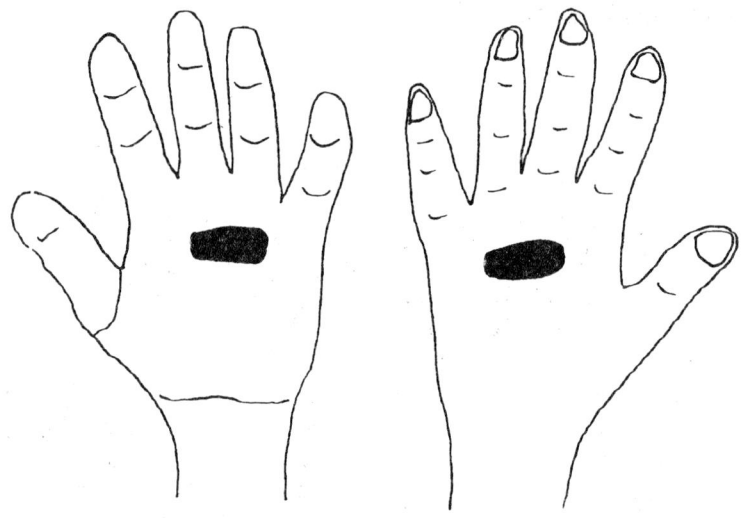

Maureen, an adolescent girl, suffered from pain in the chest during inhalation. After an course of four daily eight-minute treatments, the pain disappeared - as did the acne that had plagued her.

43

Point number 43 is situated below the pinkie on the upper part of both surfaces of the **left** hand only.

Pressure on this point is helpful in cases of anemia, digestive problems, inflammations, and nosebleeds.

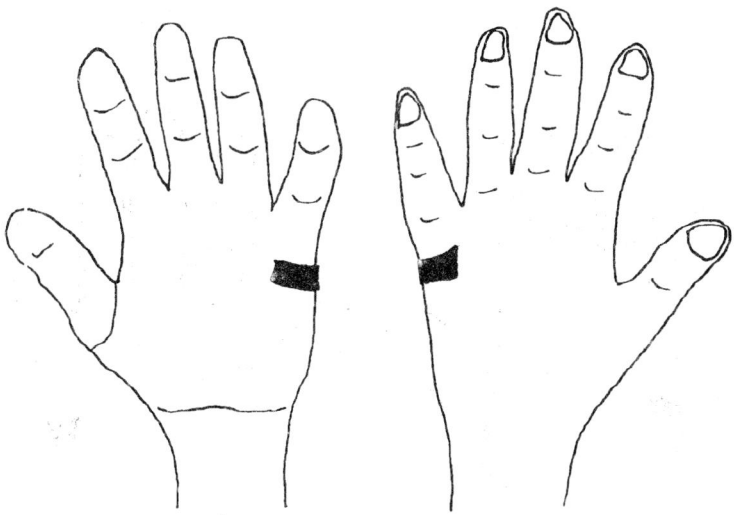

Danny was considered the weakling of the neighborhood. He never felt good, suffered from nosebleeds and from a variety of aches and pains, required special foods, and never took part in anything. A long-term course of six daily five-minute treatments curbed the nosebleeds and enabled Danny to enjoy a much wider variety of foods. He began to participate in games with the gang, and stopped suffering from various ailments as well as from the feeling of heaviness that had always encumbered him.

44

Point number 44 is situated approximately in the middle of the palm (slightly higher) beneath the pinkie on both surfaces of the **right** hand.

Pressure on this point is effective in treating digestive problems, hepatitis, liver infections, anger, and mental tension.

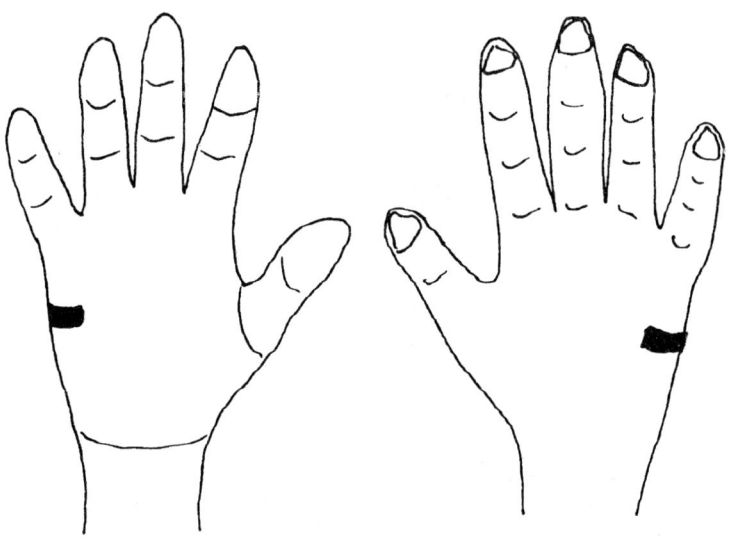

Beth was having a hard time recovering from a liver infection, so she underwent a course of four daily nine-minute treatments. She reported a significant improvement in her condition after a few days of treatment.

45

Point number 45 is situated approximately in the middle of the palm (slightly below) on the pinkie side, exactly beneath point number 44, on both surfaces of the **right** hand.

Pressure on this point helps in cases of pains in the gall bladder and gallstones, and defective digestion of fats.

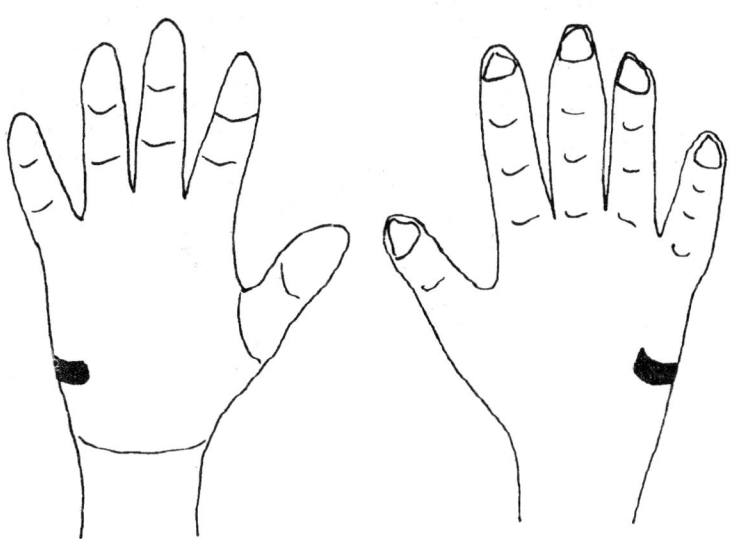

Michelle suffered from acute attacks of abdominal pains. An ultrasound examination revealed gallstones. Four daily nine-minute treatments helped relieve the pain.

The Back of the Hand
46

Point number 46 is situated on the back of the hand, in the middle, in the area beneath the index finger.

Pressure on this point alleviates rheumatic pains in the hand joints and the shoulders, and eases pains in the muscles and bones of the shoulder region.

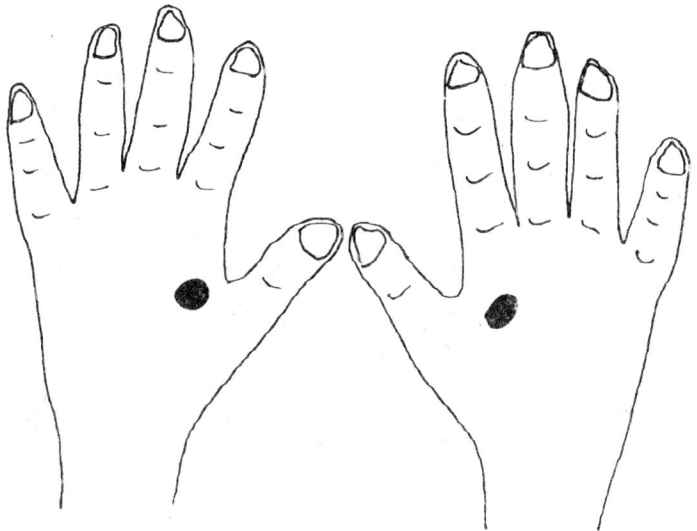

Gideon embarked on a whole lot of athletic activities simultaneously without the prerequisite physical preparation. After a few work-outs, he experienced acute pain in the shoulder region. Three daily 10-minute treatments over a relatively short period relieved the pain, and now Alan works out in moderation, according to his level of fitness.

47

Point number 47 is the continuation of point number 46, and is situated below it.

Pressure on this point provides relief in cases of tension and pain in the back and shoulder blades.

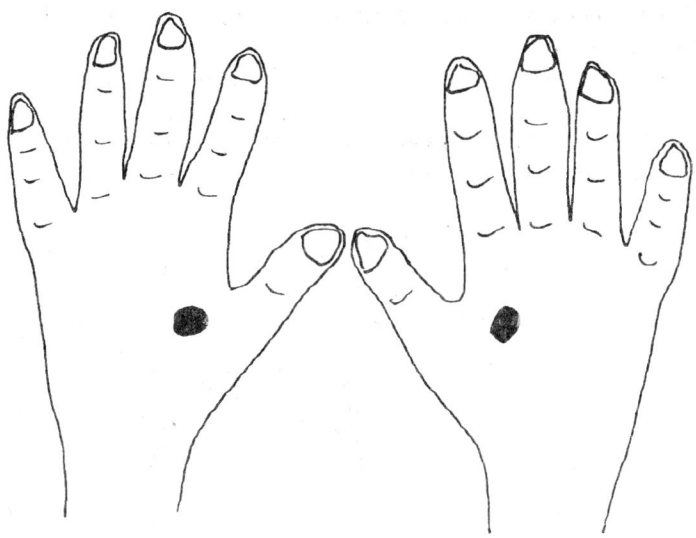

Diana, a junior high-school student, complained of pain in the region of the shoulder blades. The pain disappeared after a short period of two daily five-minute treatments. At the same time, Diana made an effort to sit correctly and hold her head erect, and the pain did not return.

48

Point number 48 comprises two strips on the back of **both** hands, which create a triangle between the index finger and the thumb. One strip begins at the base of the index finger and descends in a straight line to the point where the bones of the thumb connect to those of the index finger, and the second descends from the point where the thumb is connected to the hand, to the point where it meets the first strip.

Pressure on these points is effective in cases of back pains, headaches, menstrual pains, insufficient production of mother's milk, digestive problems, hemorrhoids, and problems with posture.

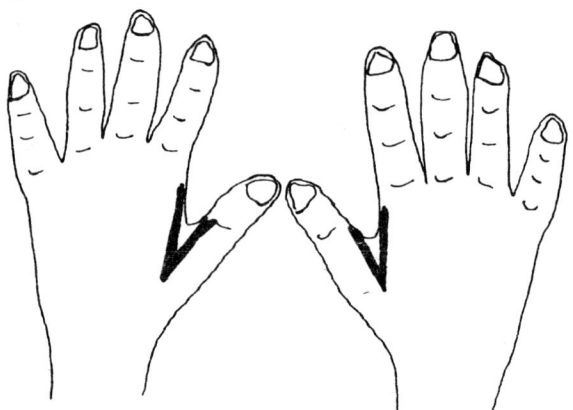

After the birth of her first child, Julia suffered from anemia and insufficient milk production. Six daily ten-minute treatments were very helpful in alleviating these problems, as well as in curing Julia's abdominal pains, headaches and hemorrhoids.

49

Point number 49 is situated below the index finger in the region where the bones of the thumb and index finger connect at the back of both hands.

Pressure on this point alleviates all lower back pains as well as pains in the muscles of the buttocks.

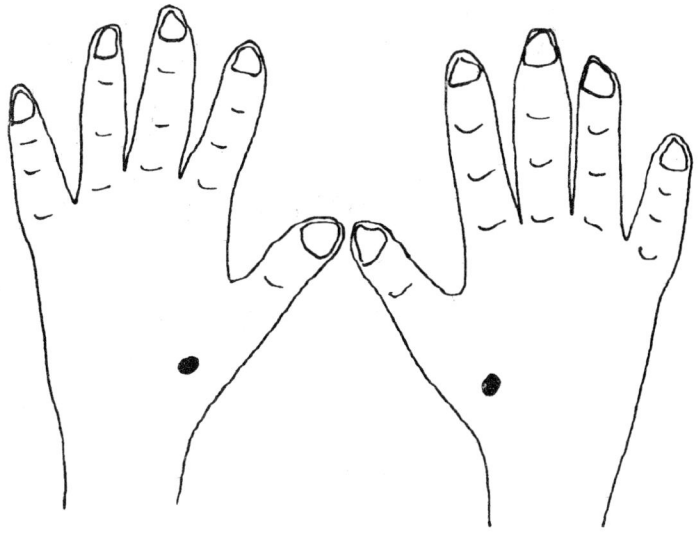

After driving his bus for hours on end every day, Harry had constant lower back pains. Now, six times a day between trips, he administers 10-minute massage treatments to the appropriate point on his hand, and this enables him to continue driving without pain.

50

Point number 50 is situated above point number 49.

Pressure on point number 50 alleviates lower back pains, as well as pains in the hip region and in the muscles of the lower abdomen.

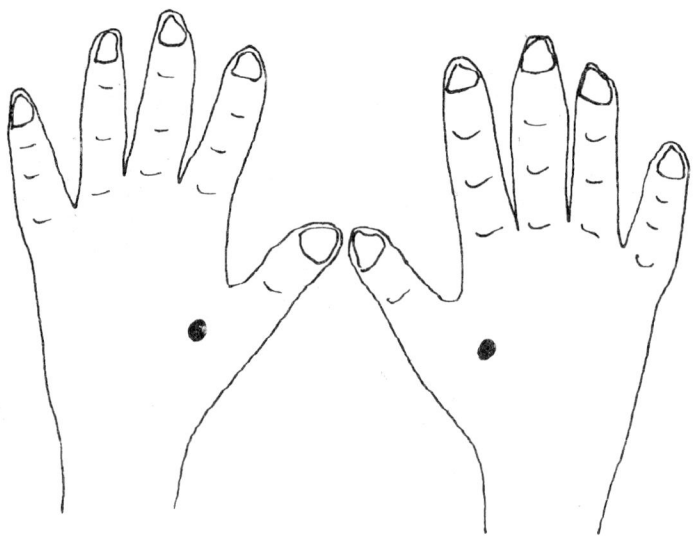

Anna suffered from constant pains in the region around and below the hip. She stopped wearing high heels and tried to stabilize her posture, but to no avail. After a course of three daily five-minute treatments for six months, she could wear shoes with medium heels, and reported a significant improvement in her condition.

The Palm/The Root of the Hand
51

Point number 51 is situated beneath the pinkie above the root of the palm on both hands.

Pressure on this point is effective with "caught" or tense muscles and pains in the sciatic nerve (at the back of the legs).

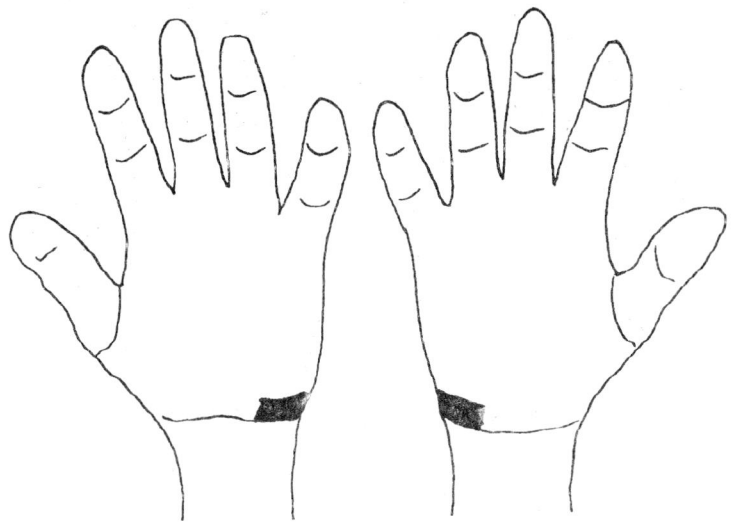

Ron suffered from almost constantly "caught" leg muscles, a problem which bothered him greatly both professionally and socially. After learning to massage the appropriate point for five minutes three times a day, Ron is considering taking up power walking ...

The Root of the Hand
52

Point number 52 is a narrow strip across the root of the palm.

Pressure on this strip is effective in treating anal pain and hemorrhoids.

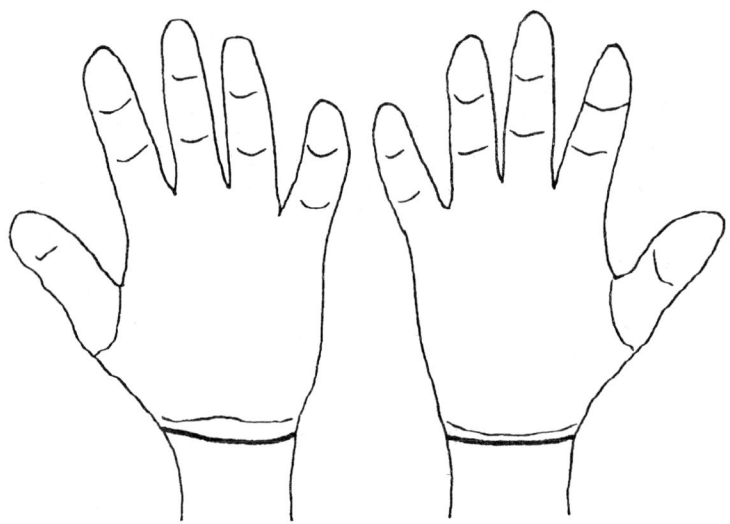

Jim was tormented by bleeding hemorrhoids. When rubber rings and various ointments proved useless, I recommended exercise, fiber-rich health food, and eight daily nine-minute massages of the appropriate point. Now three daily five-minute treatments suffice for Jim to prevent the recurrence of the unpleasant condition.

53

Point number 53 is a horizontal strip situated at the root of the back of the hand.

Pressure on this strip is effective against itching, eczema, and painful swollen glands in the groin region.

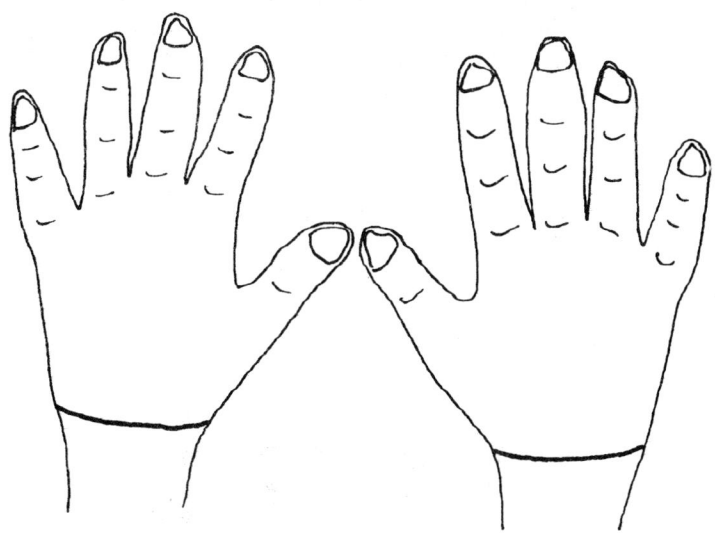

Al broke out in painful sores in the groin that hindered his everyday activities; trousers made of certain fabrics caused him to itch diabolically. Neither wearing boxer shorts nor giving up his jeans helped (the sores just didn't go away. He administered six daily eight-minute self-treatments until the sores disappeared.

54/55/56/57/58

Points number 58, 56 and 57 are situated below the base of the inner side of the palms (i.e. on the thumb side), with point 58 close to the root of the palm, point 56 beneath it, and point 57 beneath point 56.

Points number 54 and 55 are situated below the base of the outer side of the palms (i.e. on the pinkie side), with point 54 opposite point 56 and point 55 opposite point 57.

Pressure on these points is effective in cases of fertility problems, glandular diseases, and sexual dysfunction.

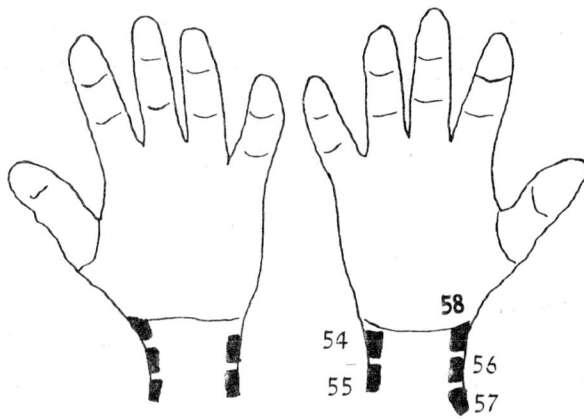

Both Brad and Mel came to the clinic with problems of premature ejaculation. Denise complained of irregular periods, while Tina had never experienced an orgasm in her life. Each patient was shown how to administer a suitable massage to the appropriate point at the base of the palm. The number of daily treatments ranged from three to six daily treatments of six to eight minutes each. At their half-yearly check-up, the patients reported an improvement in their conditions.

REFLEXOLOGY OF THE FOOT

1

Point number 1 is situated in the center of the lower part of both big toes.

Treatment of this point is effective in cases of: eczema, rheumatism, blocked arteries, lack of sugar, impotence, general physical ailments, multiple sclerosis, growth problems, problems of metabolism, and regulation of internal glandular secretion.

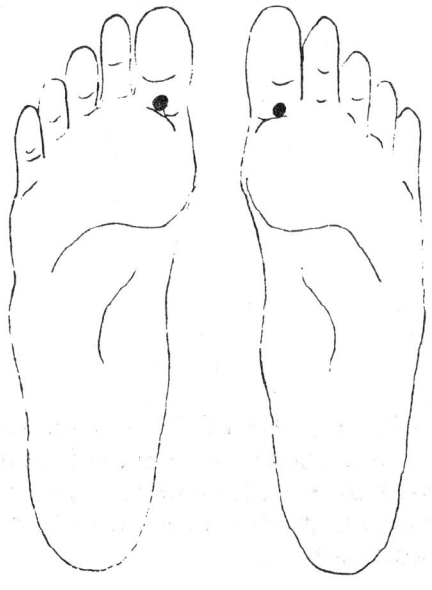

Robert suffered from unexplained pains all over his body. After undergoing extensive medical tests and taking every possible medication, he came to the clinic, where we began to treat point number 1. When his condition has stabilized and the pains have decreased, we will identify the source of the pain and administer specific treatment.

2

Point number 2 includes the outer edges of the toes of both feet.

Treatment of these points will relieve cases of stroke and sinusitis.

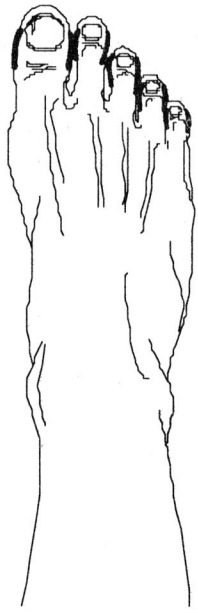

Dana suffered from frequent and severe sinusitis attacks, causing her acute suffering as well as many missed work days. After receiving treatment, she learned how to massage the tips of her toes (and the sinusitis has never come back.

3

Point number 3 is situated in the joints connecting the toes to the foot, on both surfaces of the feet.

Treatment of these points is helpful for problems of metabolism, dry skin, cholesterol, growth and development, low calcium level, spasms, sore throats, tonsillitis, and stiff necks. Toothache must be treated in the area on the upper surface of the toes.

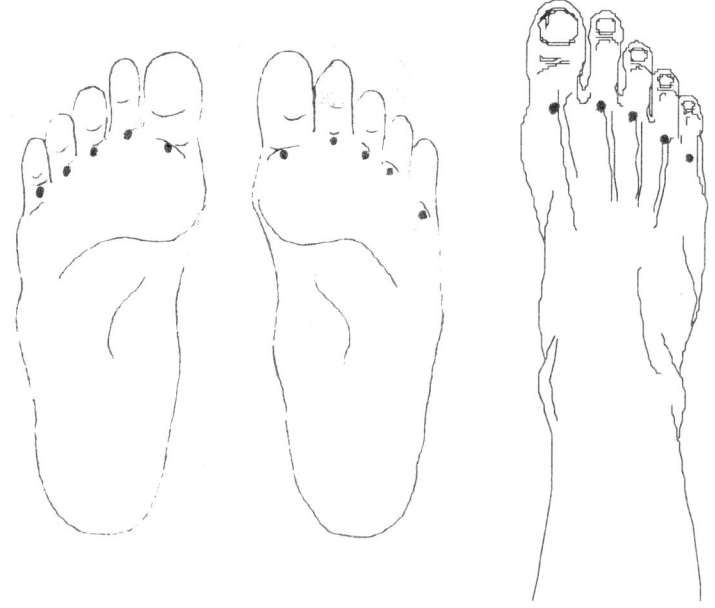

At 13, Neil was short for his age. Medical tests revealed that his thyroid gland was malfunctioning. Before embarking upon conventional treatment, he came to the clinic and was administered treatment consisting of pressure on the appropriate point. His physicians reported an improvement in his condition.

4

Point number 4 is situated in the place where the big toe joins the foot, on the side and underside of both feet, and corresponds to the neck vertebrae.

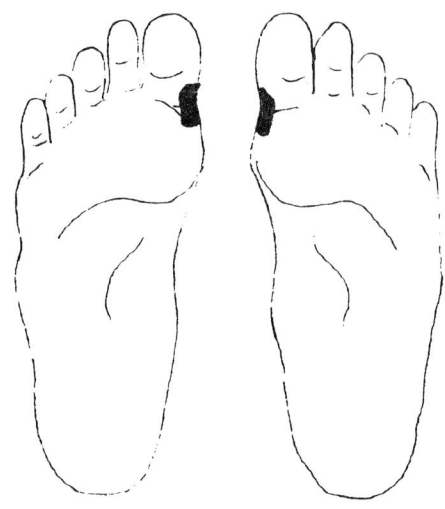

Sidney, a senior manager in a hi-tech company, suffered from agonizing neck pains. After conventional treatment did not help, he consulted with a reflexologist, who taught him how to massage point number 4. His pains disappeared.

5

Point number 5 is a small triangle situated below the join of the big toe in the direction of the ball of the foot, and corresponds to the thymus gland.

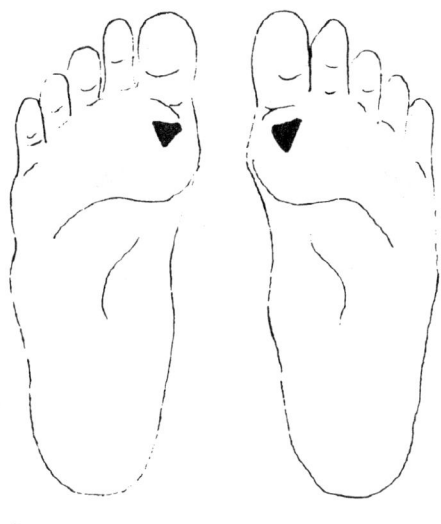

(This point is used by conventional physicians, who recommend massaging it in conjunction with treatment with conventional medication. Consult with your personal physician if you have any problem with glands.)

6

Point number 6 is a strip situated below the second, third, fourth and baby toes, on the soles of both feet.

Treatment of this point is effective in cases of: vertigo, temporary loss of balance, inner ear infections, fainting spells, eye strain, and tinnitus (ringing in the ears).

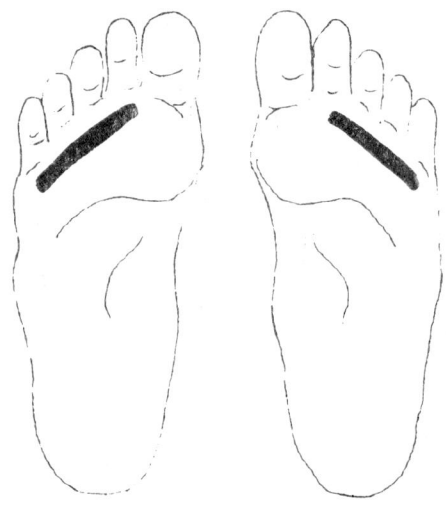

Laura suffered from a constant ringing in her ears which bothered her and prevented her from leading a normal life. After undergoing treatment in the clinic, she learned to massage the appropriate point – and the ringing stopped.

7

Point number 7 is situated along the length of the inner side of the feet.

Pressure on this point is effective in treating multiple sclerosis, which is a chronic disease of the central nervous system, destroying the capacity for voluntary movement.

(Point number 7 is also divided into four secondary strips, each of which corresponds to a particular area:

7a. The neck vertebrae

7b. The chest vertebrae

7c. The vertebrae in the hip region: treatment of point 7c is helpful in the case of shingles.

7d. The tailbone, the rectum and the anus: treatment of point 7d is effective in cases of constipation and hemorrhoids.)

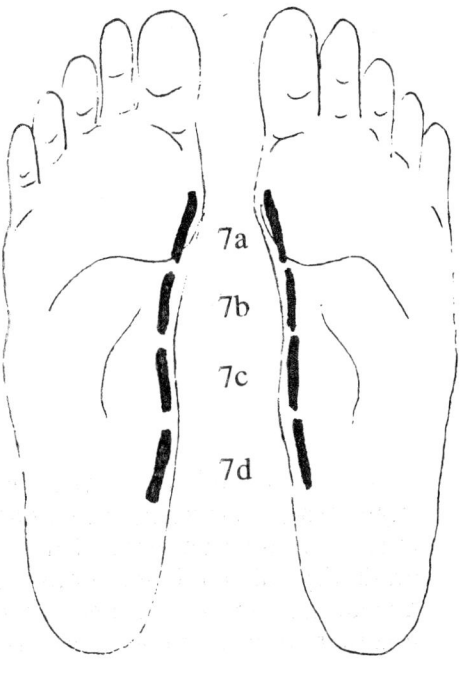

Gina had been involved in a serious accident. After a series of operations, it was still very difficult for her to walk. She became progressively weaker, and often complained of a feeling resembling paralysis in her limbs. She required an especially lengthy course of treatment, but today she functions almost normally.

8

Point number 8 is situated below the baby toe at the outer side of both feet.

Treatment of this point alleviates pains in the arms.

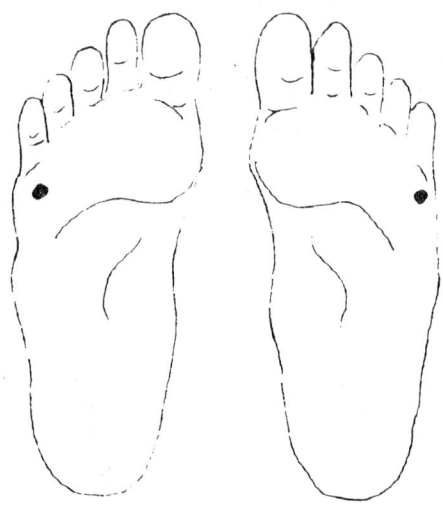

Alex suffered from acute pains in the muscles of his right arm, stemming, apparently, from overuse of the muscle. After treatment of the appropriate point, the pain gradually subsided, and today Alex is aware of how much he can use the muscle, and when he needs to administer a treatment in order to prevent a painful attack.

9

Point number 9 is situated on the soles of both feet below the baby toe, in the region of the ball of the foot.

Treatment of this point is effective for pains in the shoulders and shoulder blades.

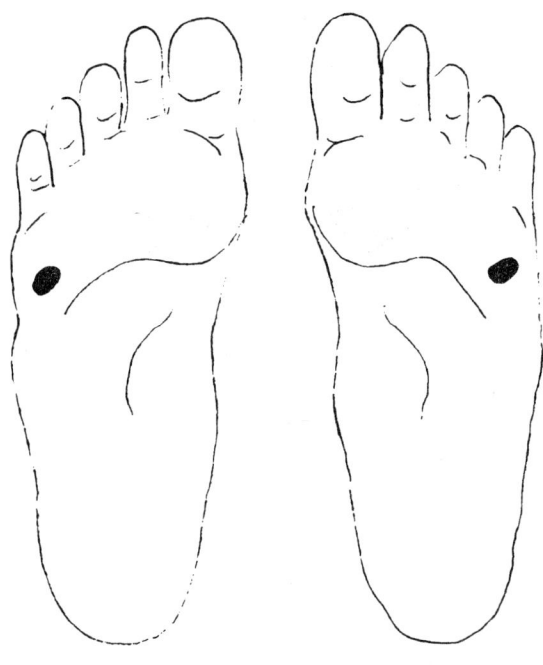

10

Point number 10 is situated on the large ball of both feet, below the big toe and the three toes next to it.

On the **right** foot, the point corresponds to the lungs. On the **left** foot, the point corresponds to heart and lungs.

Treatment of these points is helpful in cases of colds (infections of the mucous membranes of the nose and throat.

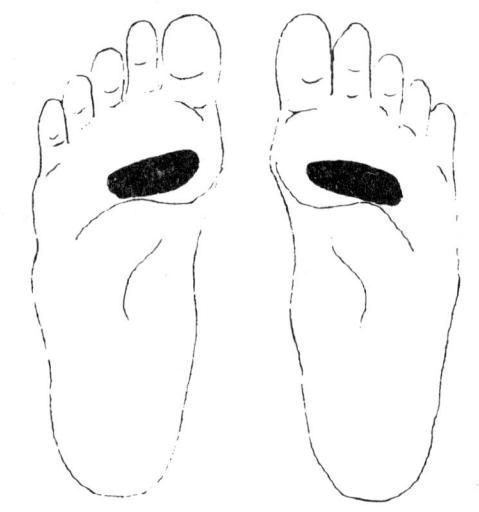

Since childhood, Lee suffered from recurring colds. When she could no longer bear this situation, she underwent treatment on a regular basis. For the last two winters, she has not had a cold.

11

Point number 11 traverses the soles below the balls of the feet. (The strip constitutes the boundary between the arch and the ball.)

Treatment of this point is helpful for: acne, rheumatism, asthma, laryngitis, shortness of breath, problems associated with the heart muscle, ulcer, heartburn. In the case of a hernia, only the point in the area below the big toe on the right foot should be pressed.

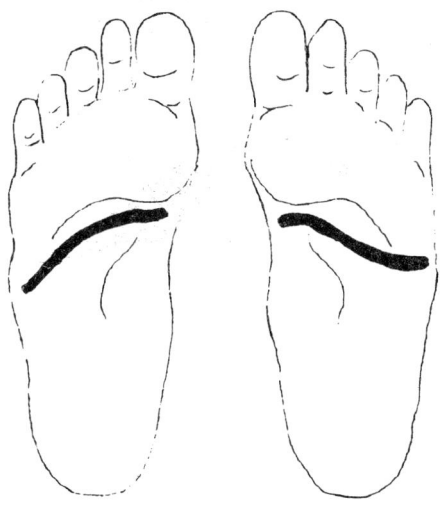

The Robinsons moved from a dry area to a humid one. A few days later, Mrs. Robinson experienced difficulty in breathing, which did not subside, but instead worsened. She came to the clinic and underwent treatment on a daily basis until her condition improved.

12

Point number 12 is situated on the sole of the **left** foot beneath the big toe, at the beginning of the arch, and on the sole of the **right** foot on the whole area of the arch, from one end to the other.

Pressure on this point is effective in treating liver problems.

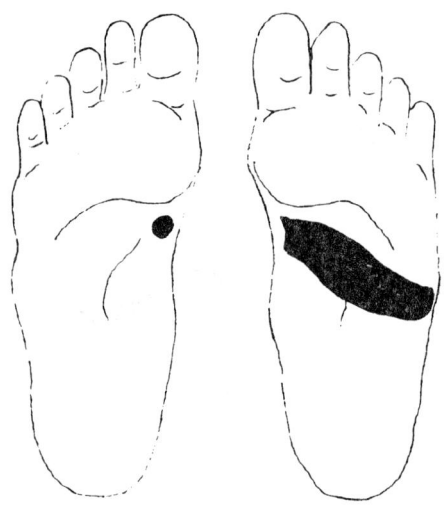

Julie came down with hepatitis. In order to speed up her recuperation, she received treatment of point number 12, which was extremely helpful.

13

Point number 13 is situated on the sole of the **left** foot in the region of the arch beneath the three middle toes.

Treatment of this point helps treat ulcers and digestive problems.

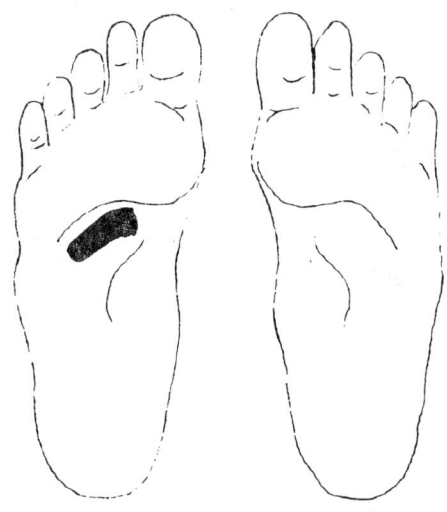

Since he was a teenager, Steve suffered from a stomach ulcer, and refrained from eating certain foods which, in his opinion, had a deleterious effect on his condition. After an especially acute attack, he came to the clinic, where he learned the appropriate point for administering self-treatment. The frequency and acuteness of the attacks began to decrease, and with the correct diet, Steve would soon be able to forget the problems that had plagued him for so many years.

14

Point number 14 is situated on the sole of the **left** foot in the region of the arch between the fourth and baby toes.

Treatment of this point helps in cases of infection and the need to control the number of red blood cells.

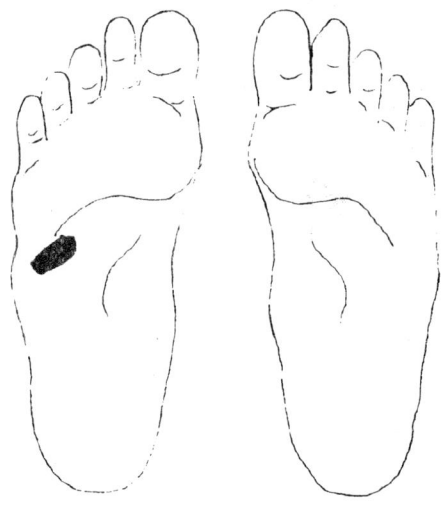

Billie suffered from a problematic wound on her leg. After a long time, when the wound still had not healed, but instead exuded pus, she came to the clinic (actually for the treatment of some other problem entirely. When by chance I noticed the swollen area with the wound in the middle of it, I offered to help her, and today only a tiny scar remains.

15

Point number 15 is situated in the region of the arch of the **right** foot, between the fourth and baby toes.

Treatment of this point is helpful in cases of problems of digestion of fats, and pains in the gall bladder.

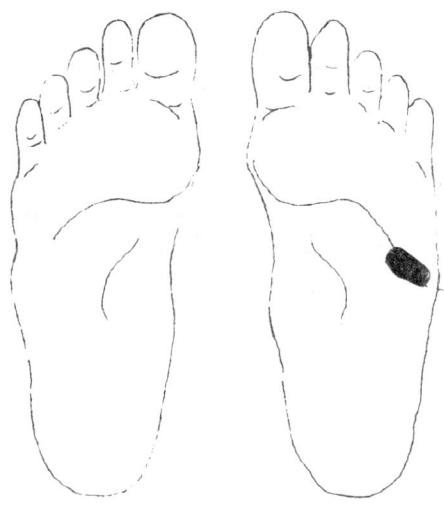

After having her gallbladder surgically removed because of gallstones, Cindy suffered from pains in that region every time she ate food containing fat. With our guidance, she learned to cut down on fatty foods, and also to locate and massage the appropriate point.

16

Point number 16 is situated at the very highest point of the arch, beneath the big toe on the soles of both feet.

Treatment of this point is effective in maintaining the correct sugar levels in the blood, mental alertness, and a high energy level.

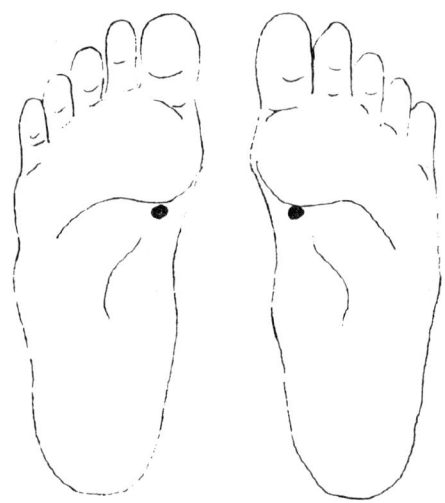

In Pamela's family, there was a history of diabetes. When Pamela felt a lack of energy, a constant thirst, and a certain degree of weakness, she identified the signs and came to the clinic where she learned to treat herself before her condition deteriorated.

17

Point number 17 traverses the center of the soles of both feet, from the inner side to beneath the middle of the baby toe.

Pressure on this point is effective for treating digestive problems and colitis (inflammation of the large intestine).

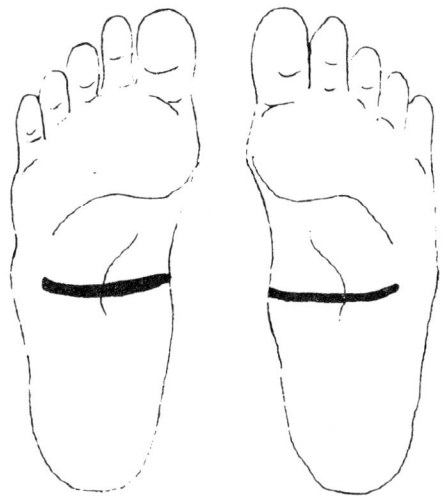

Pat suffered from a serious problem of stomach-aches and flatulence that medical treatment did not succeed in curing. Administering a massage to point number 17 solved her problem.

18

Point number 18 is situated on the sole of the **left** foot, beneath the middle of the baby toe, and joins up with point number 17.

Pressure on point number 18 helps in cases of digestive problems and colitis.

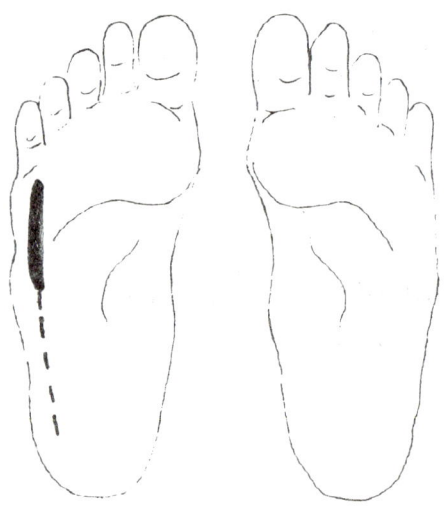

Dan, an officer in the military, suffered from severe stomach pains. After treatment with medications did not get to the root of the problem, he learnt to administer a daily massage of point number 18. His stomach pains eased up and almost disappeared.

19

Point number 19 is situated on the sole of the **right** foot, beneath the baby toe, up to where the heel starts.

Treatment of point number 19 is effective in cases of digestive problems and colitis (like point number 18).

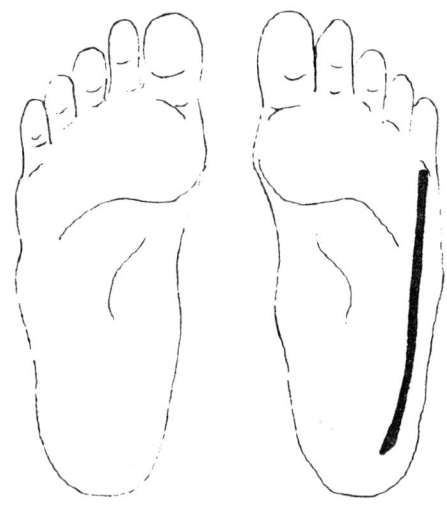

Rhona suffered from a problem of constant intestinal cramps. A reflexologist in her clinic prepared an inner sole for her with protruding areas that massaged point number 19 while she walked. The cramps disappeared.

20/21

Point number 20 is situated on the **left** heel, between the end of point number 18 and the opposite end.

Treatment of this point is helpful in cases of digestive problems and intestinal inflammations.

Point number 21 is situated on the heel of the **right** foot, at the end of strip number 19. Treatment of this point has a similar effect to that of point number 20.

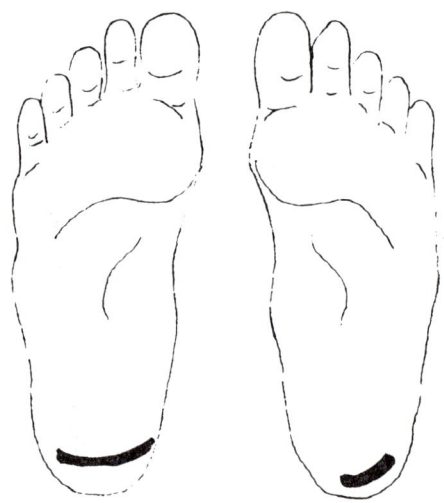

Jessica suffered from acute constipation accompanied by abdominal pains. She was diagnosed as having "lazy bowel syndrome," and resigned herself to having to use digestive stimulants for the rest of her life. I suggested appropriate treatment along with a diet based primarily on fruits and vegetables. Now she needs laxatives only on rare occasions.

22

Point number 22 is situated between the arch and the heel on the area beneath the big toe and the three next toes, on the soles of both feet.

Treatment of this point is effective in cases of digestive problems (especially in the small intestine).

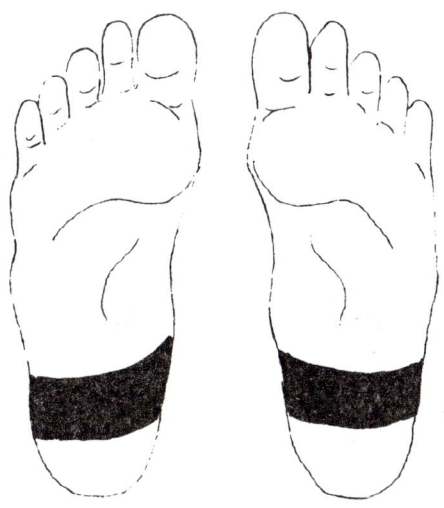

Judy suffered from attacks of vomiting and abdominal pains for no apparent reason. The situation became so acute that she was afraid to eat or drink anything. Routine treatment caused the symptoms to disappear.

23

Point number 23 is situated in the center of both soles.

Treatment of this point helps in cases of: excess uric acid in the blood which causes gout, kidney and urinary tract infections, and psoriasis.

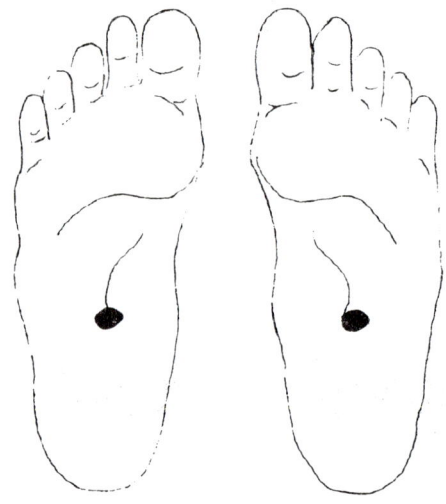

Even after Fred had completed a course of conventional treatment for a urinary tract infection, he still had pain. After a series of treatments in the clinic, the pain ceased, as did the constant urge to urinate.

24

Point number 24 is situated beneath the big toe and above point number 23 on the soles of both feet.

Treatment of point number 24 is effective in cases of: tension, endurance problems, lack of energy, infection, inflammation, allergy, hernia.

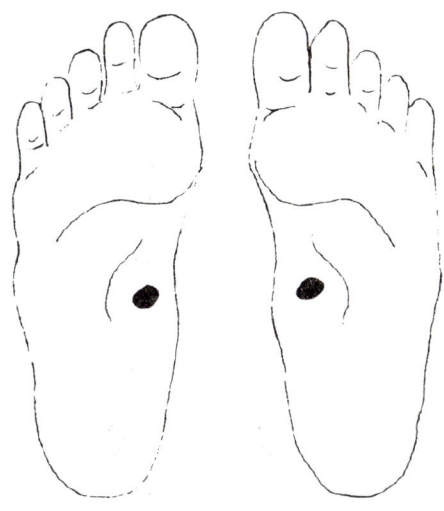

At the age of 53, Dave discovered that he was allergic to almonds. Every time he ate them, his lips would swell up, and he would feel exhausted. He cut down on his activities and began to withdraw to his home. His son brought him to the clinic, where he was finally persuaded that he was not aging quickly, and that his condition could be treated.

25

Point number 25 is situated on the inner side of both feet, at the beginning of the heel on the big toe side.

Treatment of this point helps prevent fluid retention, regulates acids, and balances the substances in the blood.

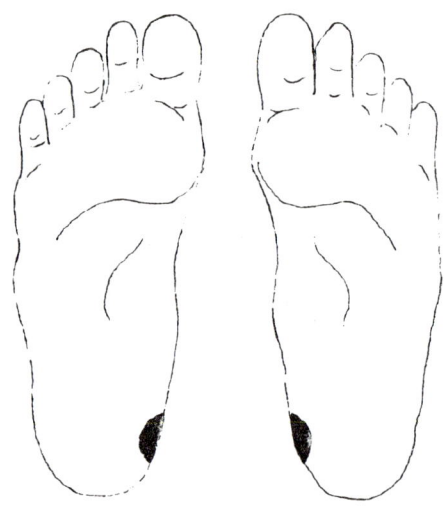

Marcy developed edema (swelling) in her feet, to the point that she could not wear any shoes. After a series of treatments, the swelling disappeared. Marcy undergoes a weekly massage in order to prevent the condition from recurring.

26

Point number 26 appears as a strip along the heel on the inner side of both feet.

Treatment of this point helps alleviate pains resulting from problems in the tailbone.

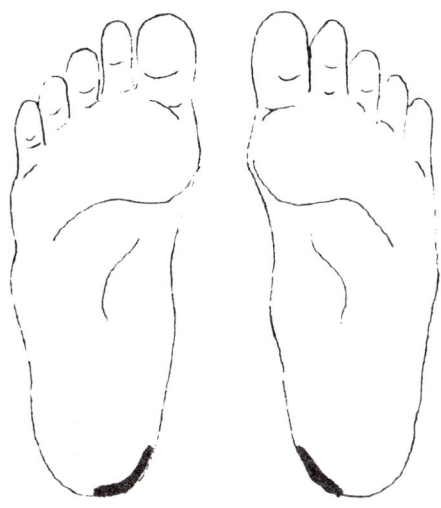

Jake suffered from agonizing back pains, which originated in the lower back. A weekly massage of point number 26 administered by a reflexologist relieved the pain, and Jake resumed a normal life.

27

Point number 27 is situated in the rear area of the heels of both feet.

Treatment of this point is effective in cases of constipation which is a side-effect of stress, and pressure on the lower back.

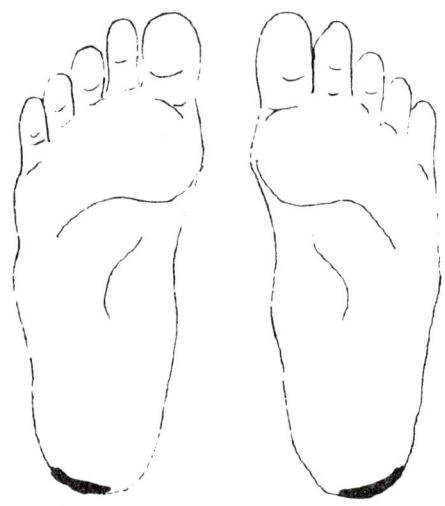

Joel was a soldier doing a tour of duty in a hostile country. He spent most of his time patrolling dangerous urban areas. After suffering from constipation for six months – without knowing why, as his diet was regular and balanced, and he did not experience nausea or stomach pains – I treated him, and today he knows how to massage his heels and prevent an unpleasant feeling.

28

Point number 28 is situated on the upper surface of both feet, between the big toe and the second toe, and corresponds to the lymphatic system.

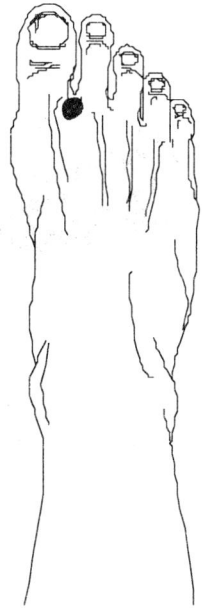

(This point must be treated **only** by a qualified physician. It is treated in cases of abnormality in the absorption or accumulation of liquids in the body.)

29

Point number 29 appears as a strip right across the top of both feet, extending from the root of the toes to halfway down the top of the foot.

Treatment of this point helps relieve muscle pain caused by a stiff neck.

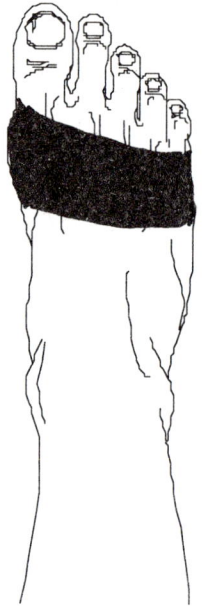

Traveling to the clinic in a taxi one day, I immediately noticed that the taxi driver's body was stiff and his movements limited. It turned out that he suffered from a painfully stiff neck. I invited him to come into the clinic, where he received "emergency treatment," and learned how to administer self-treatment during his breaks from driving.

30

Point number 30 is situated across the top of both feet, close to strip number 28.

Treatment of point number 30 is effective in cases of pains stemming from problems in the vertebrae of the middle back.

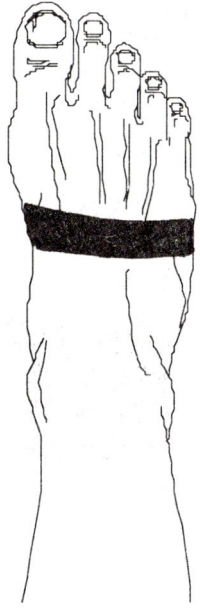

Another taxi driver arrived at the clinic, suffering from back pains. He told me that the cushions he placed behind him to support his back while driving no longer helped. Like his colleague, he was given "emergency treatment" and learned how to administer self-treatments during his breaks between fares.

31

Point number 31 appears in the middle of the upper surface of both feet, reaching the point where the foot joins the calf, around the whole foot, including the heel.

Treatment of this point is helpful in cases of pains that stem from lower back problems such as: inflammation of the large intestine, and headaches resulting from physical conditions, stress or medications.

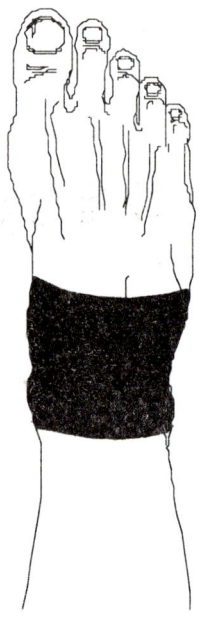

Sandra came to the clinic suffering from headaches and abdominal pains. As she was a student just before her final exams, and there was no apparent reason for her ailments other than stress, she received the appropriate treatment, and got through the exam period without being troubled by the symptoms she had reported previously.

32

Point number 32 is situated around the connecting line between the calf and the upper surface of both feet.

Treatment of this point is effective after hysterectomies, in cases of infertility, and in cases of untoward swelling in the veins (generally in the legs).

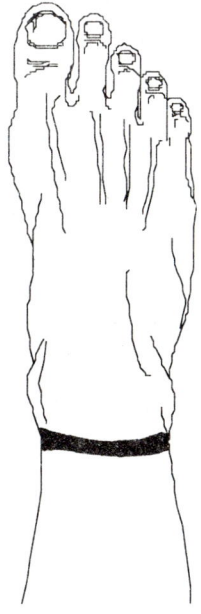

Gabriella was compelled to undergo a hysterectomy after a particularly difficult birth. Her recuperation was extremely slow, both for physical and psychological reasons. After a series of treatments, she began to feel better, and resumed her regular life style.

33

Point number 33 is situated above the heel, below the ankle bone on the inner and outer sides of both feet.

Treatment of this point is helpful in: maintaining the libido, mental alertness, physical development, hysterectomy, impotence, infertility, fluid retention, and menstrual problems.

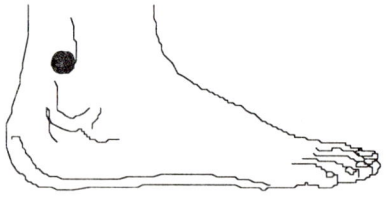

Arthur suffered from recurring inflammations of the prostate, which impaired his sexual functioning and caused pain when he urinated. Treatment of the appropriate point helped, and the condition began to disappear rapidly.

34

Point number 34 is situated above the ankle bone on the outer side of the leg.

Treatment of this point is helpful in the case of pain in the tendons in the legs.

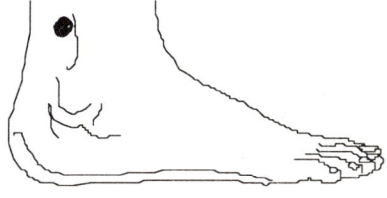

Claire had reached the point where the pain in her legs, which originated from the thigh muscle, almost prevented her from leaving her house. After a lengthy series of treatments at the clinic, she could discard the walking stick that had been her companion her over the last few months. She soon regained almost the full extent of her former ambulatory powers.

35

Point number 35 is situated on the outer side of the feet before the beginning of the heel area.

Treatment of this point is helpful in cases of pains in the lower part of the body (from the hips down) and inflammation of the veins.

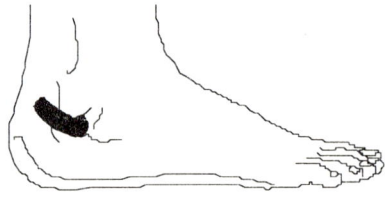

Louis, a man in his eighties, had been suffering from pains in his legs and swollen veins in his left leg for years. When he reached the point where he could no longer get out of bed and stand up, I went to the senior citizens' home where he lived and administered a series of treatments to him. Eventually he got up and resumed the social activities he had enjoyed before.